# TEN MILLION STEPS

## THE INCREDIBLE JOURNEY OF
## PAUL REESE, WHO RAN ACROSS AMERICA –
## A MARATHON A DAY FOR 124 DAYS – AT AGE 73

### By Paul Reese
### and Joe Henderson

W, th best wishes,
Paul Reese
Oct 21, 1993

First published in the United States of America in 1993 by WRS Publishing, A Division of WRS Group, Inc., 701 N. New Road, Waco, Texas 76710
Front cover photo by Kenneth Lee
Book design by Kenneth Turbeville
Jacket design by Talmage Minter

10 9 8 7 6 5 4 3 2 1

Library of Congress Cataloging-in-Publication Data

Reese, Paul.
    Ten million steps : the incredible journey of Paul Reese, who ran across America—a marathon a day for 124 days—at age 73 / by Paul Reese and Joe Henderson.
        p.        cm.
    ISBN 1-56796-014-6 : $12.95
    1. Reese, Paul. 2. Runners (Sports)—United States—Biography. 3. Aged athletes—United States—Biography. I. Henderson, Joe, 1943–   . II. Title.
GV1061. 15.R44A3 1993
796.42' 092—dc20
    [B]
                                                                    93-23186
                                                                        CIP

## TO ELAINE

*Whose support was as essential as my two legs
in making this run, and whose caring and
sharing made it one of the most enjoyable
experiences of my life.*

# Contents

# Foreword

I could hardly believe what I was reading. In fact, I had to reread it just to make sure I had read it correctly. What I read was that a 73-year-old man named Paul Reese was going to attempt a 3,200-mile run across the United States.

The distance was staggering enough, though I knew that several others had run across the country, but for a 73-year-old to even be thinking about it, let alone actually attempting it, had me shaking my head in disbelief.

At the same time, I was smiling inwardly as I thought: If he succeeds, this will be a giant step forward regarding our concepts about aging. It will awaken people in their sixties and seventies to their inherent physical capabilities. And it will be proof positive to younger people that in their sunset years they will be capable of considerably more physical activity than they previously realized, providing they regulate their lifestyles.

Reading about this projected run, and thinking about it, I decided to follow Paul's progress as he went across the country. This was an easy chore because I was on the mailing list of family and friends to whom Paul sent a progress report at 1,000 miles, 2,000 miles, and when he finished.

When I read about his splashing into the Atlantic Ocean at Hilton Head Island to culminate a 3,192-mile massive trek across the country, I felt awe and admiration for his accomplishment. Talk about role models, Paul gets my vote as the first centerfold for Modern Maturity!

As Chairman of the President's Council on Physical Fitness and Sports, I was glad to see such a strong statement made for physical fitness and for aging gracefully. Truly, the running shoe has replaced the rocking chair as a national symbol for healthy aging. The difference in cost between a pair of NIKEs or a Lifecycle and a double heart bypass can be significant!

To read *Ten Million Steps* is to step into the shoes and mind of a 73-year-old man as he runs through twelve states on his way from the Pacific Ocean in California to the Atlantic Ocean in South Carolina.

It's a highly inspirational story.

But don't get me wrong—yes, it did inspire me, but I'm not about to try to run all the way across the country. Maybe, though, when I'm 73, I'll change my mind!

ARNOLD SCHWARZENEGGER

# *Preface*

Other runners had already done what Paul Reese did. Dozens of them had crossed the United States on foot, many of them taking less time than he took, some doing it in races, and some for money-making causes or as self-promotional stunts.

The most remarkable thing about Paul Reese's journey of national and personal discovery was what he DIDN'T do. He didn't try to break any records or raise any money. He didn't act as a paid spokesman for seniors or cancer patients. He didn't want to draw attention to himself or even plan initially to publish this book.

Reese kept his intentions quiet partly to protect himself from skeptics who would have said, "It can't be done at your age," and from friends who might have said, "It shouldn't be done in your health."

The runner from Auburn, California, would turn 73 the week his journey was to begin in the spring of 1990. Articles of faith in this sport are that recovery from big efforts slows down with age and that a senior athlete should attempt only one or two marathons each year. Reese planned to run a marathon EACH DAY for four straight months.

Reese also was just coming off a cancer scare. A cancerous prostate had been diagnosed less than three years earlier, and apparently had been treated successfully with radiation. But you could never tell what chain reactions the stress of this run might set off.

So he plotted the journey quietly. He organized it without sponsorship, without a support crew other than his wife Elaine, and without seeking any publicity.

He didn't even tell me, and I've known Paul for 25 years. We've run hundreds of miles together in races. He knew I, as a running writer, couldn't be trusted to keep his secret, so he kept it to himself.

I didn't learn what he was doing until he'd done it. Even then, the news didn't come from him but from a gossip column in a San Francisco newspaper.

Another year passed before I learned that Paul had written a book-length manuscript en route. Each night, he'd captured in his journal the thoughts and observations from his day on the back roads of America. He'd meant this only as a personal record book.

"I wanted it to record the heat of battle, and not write it later and have actuality changed by reflection," he told me in a P.S. to a letter on another subject. He made me work to get a copy of the journal.

"Just don't advertise it," he warned. "I don't want to get in the book-supply business."

The manuscript somehow found its way to Dr. Wayman Spence, who IS in the business of supplying books. You now hold the book Reese didn't originally write for publication. The WRS editors and I slimmed it down for print. But it retains all of the immediacy and intimacy of Paul's heat-of-battle report.

Like all extended battles, this one mixes anticipation with dread, adventure with exhaustion, triumph with setback, confidence with doubt, joy with relief. Like all difficult journeys, this one shows the traveler where he has gone and what he saw there—and, even more, it shows him who he is and how far he can push himself.

JOE HENDERSON,
*Runner's World* Magazine

# Author's Note

I am the oldest person to run across the United States. This is an account of that 3,192-mile run at age 73.

Each day as I went across the country, a different drama played out. Each day was awash with suspense, action, and the conflict of dealing with weather, traffic, and bad roads.

As the curtain went up on each new day, we never quite knew what would develop before we came to rest at the next overnight stopping place. At the end of the day, we reviewed that day and geared for the next.

Thus, we lived one day at a time. To us the adventure was a play with 124 acts.

The best way I can tell our story is to unfold it day by day just as it happened. The best way for a reader to step into my shoes is to relive the trek day by day.

The strength, the authenticity, the bloodline of this book is that each day was written when and as it happened. And here it stands, unique among other books about foot-crossings of the USA. All others were written after the fact.

Recollection has a way of tampering with what actually happened. As time passes, experiences get easier, get harder, get exaggerated, get downplayed.

When people hear about the run, too many of them think of it as just a run. Ten million footsteps.

Central to the book, of course, is the challenge of putting one foot in front of the other ten million times. But the experience goes beyond running, to other meanings, other messages.

First, it makes a statement about aging. People over 65 don't belong in rocking chairs. They are capable of more physical activity than they realize. Who would have believed that a 73-year-old could run across the USA?

Second, the book shows that I am not blessed with super genes. I've been bothered by a bad back, and I've been treated for prostate cancer. The lesson here is that in life you dance the best you can with the music being played.

Third, the run reflects the importance of determination and resolve in accomplishing a goal. Elaine and I never wavered in our resolve to go from Pacific to Atlantic, and that resolve was cardinal to our success.

Fourth, much of this book revolves around two people

working harmoniously to accomplish a goal, because we were already close and the experience brought us closer. To borrow a phrase from a Marine classmate who read the manuscript, this is "a tribute to a marriage."

Finally, there is even a message of spirituality in these pages, because our path across the country was paved with lots of prayers. Both Elaine and I recognize that we were successful only by the grace of God.

We feel lucky to have had this experience. Very lucky.

There are so many people to thank for getting this book to press that I stumble at where to begin. Maybe right at the top would be a good idea. That means with Dr. Wayman R. Spence, whose vision and quest it is to bring a series of inspirational stories to readers.

Next, Joe Henderson merits recognition for his writing magic in taking my bulky 400-page journal and shaping it into the enticing prose that follows in these pages.

Thanks from both Joe and me to Margaret Leary and Terri Johnson, our editors at WRS Group. Their expertise and guidance, their tidying of the manuscript, and their forbearance with the foibles of runners (at least this one) are appreciated.

Then I'd like to thank all the friends who, in essays sprinkled throughout this book, wrote kind words about me. I'll introduce them as their writing appears.

However, one rates special mention here. I thank George Billingsley for his companionship during the first 1,300 miles that we ran together. I praise him for the courage and tenacity he displayed while battling injuries before and after we parted.

I thank my son Mark Reese and his trusty Leica for some of the photos in the book.

Bowed by many years and battered by some physical infirmities, I've often stood in need of "patching" to keep running in my sunset years. The doctors who keep me going are Loren Blickenstaff, Frank Boutin, Elliott Eisenbud, Gilbert Lang, and Erby Satter. I thank each one of them and implore them to maintain their high level of skills. I'll be back!

And of course, the entire operation would have been a mission with little meaning, if not mission impossible—without my wife Elaine. That being so, I thank her above all.

PAUL REESE
Auburn, California

# Prologue

The idea of running across the USA first dawned on me in 1968 while reading Don Shepherd's book, *My Run Across the United States*. Four years earlier, at age 48, this South African had run his 3,200 miles in 73 days—with his only support coming from the pack that he carried. My reaction to his book was, "I've gotta try this someday."

"Someday" turned out to be 22 years later. Two reasons: First, this adventure would take me four months, and I needed to be retired to leave home for that long. Second, Shepherd was more of an adventurer than I.

He ran alone, but I needed a pit crew. The logical choice was my wife, Elaine, who had crewed for me in many races over the years. The problem was, though I was retired and free to go by my retirement year of 1981, Elaine was still working full time and unavailable for a trip of this length.

Then she announced in late 1989 that she planned to retire the following March. I suggested that, if we did a transcontinental run together (her pit-crewing, me running), she could see the country in slow motion and at the same time wipe her job out of her mind. She agreed, with two stipulations: that we buy a new motor home for the trip, and that I buy her a black Labrador puppy when we returned home.

We took the first step in our planning and purchased a Mallard Sprinter 20-foot motor home. It has all the comforts of home: gas range and oven, refrigerator, dinette, shower, commode, running water, heat, air conditioner, double bed. As part of our preparation over the next few months, we took the Mallard on several short trips so Elaine could get used to handling it.

We decided the run would start in April 1990. For several months leading up to it, I ran no races—to reduce the risk of injury—but concentrated on long, slow runs. Fifteen miles was my maximum distance.

I took many of these runs with George Billingsley, who thrives on ultrarunning. Exposure to this exciting venture became too much for George, and he volunteered to join me on the transcon run. His wife, Georgia, would serve as his pit crew with two stipulations of her own: they would purchase a motor home, and she would take their three cats along.

Because George had business obligations to attend to, he left the logistical planning to Elaine and me. The first question we had to answer: Should we cover as much distance as we could in as short a time as possible, or see the country in slow motion?

The choice was easy. We agreed that our first consideration was to enjoy, and that enjoying and learning what we could along the way would take precedence over stacking up mileage each day.

From the books I'd read about other transcontinental runs (Don Shepherd's, Bruce Tulloh's *Four Million Footsteps*, and Jim Shapiro's *Meditations from the Breakdown Lane*), I concluded that these runners were primarily concerned with time and distance covered each day. Scenery and identifying with the country were secondary to them. Elaine and I resolved that this would not happen to us.

We decided that the time spent running each day was not a major concern. If we wanted to linger in the motor home and visit on a pit stop, we would. If we wanted to stop and play tourist, we would. We recognized that the push for time would not dictate everything we did.

We also agreed that we should have a daily goal for distance, and that the distance should be somewhat challenging but not far enough to preclude some recreational time after the day's run had ended. Elaine and I differed on what it should be. She favored 15 to 20 miles, while I wanted 25 to 26 miles. She went along with my choice because I was doing the running.

Elaine also let me have my way on another important consideration. I would attempt the entire run without taking a day off. Sure, I would have welcomed a day off every week and enjoyed the recreational time. But I felt that this rest and recuperation time would dilute the point I was trying to prove—that senior citizens have more potential for physical activity than they and others realize.

As much as possible, we would seek back roads. This would result in the trek being longer than a more direct route along major highways. We also planned to avoid metropolitan areas on the approximately 3,200-mile route from the Pacific to the Atlantic.

The day before we were to leave home, Elaine and I were finishing breakfast when the phone rang. Elaine answered it, then handed the phone to me and said with a snicker, "It's Anna, calling for Arnold Schwarzenegger."

Elaine thought someone was attempting a joke. But I knew the call was for real. I had written to congratulate him on being named chairman of the President's Council on Physical Fitness and Sports. At the same time, I had humorously suggested that, with his newly found responsibility for fitness, he should refrain from posing for pictures with a cigar in his mouth.

Schwarzenegger said on the phone, "The cigar pictures were for publicity. I rarely smoke." He also said he liked my sense of humor and wished me good luck on the run.

I thought that phone conversation was the end of it. But the next day, just before we left home, a large floral arrangement arrived with a note that read, "Good luck on your massive trek—Arnold Schwarzenegger." Besides being a thoughtful gesture, it was a terrific send-off.

# Overview of California

## April 21 to May 1, 1990 — 260.3 total miles

| Day | Overnight | Miles | Notes |
| --- | --- | --- | --- |
| 1 | Duncan Mills | 5.4 | Started RUNXUSA at Jenner, CA |
| 2 | Santa Rosa | 26.1 | began 26-mile-a-day routine |
| 3 | Saint Helena | 26.2 | |
| 4 | near Winters | 26.9 | |
| 5 | West Sacramento | 26.5 | |
| 6 | Plymouth | 31.0 | |
| 7 | Sacramento | 17.8 | ran one segment in High Sierra |
| 8 | Plymouth | 31.1 | started Slice 100-K race |
| 9 | near Hams Stn. | 31.1 | finished Slice 100-K race |
| 10 | near Woodfords | 25.1 | crossed Carson Pass in snow, temperature dipped to 22 with winds 40 to 50 MPH |

(first 13.2 miles in California on Day 11)

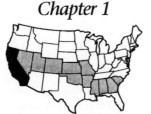

## Chapter 1

# *California, Here We Go*

California would be many things: a beginning, a farewell, and a test. It would be unlike any other state because it would be both old and new.

Old because I was born and raised here, returned here after military service, worked here as a school administrator (in Sacramento) and am now retired here (in Auburn). My three children live here. We'd say goodbye to family and friends here.

In another sense, California would be new. The run would begin at Jenner-by-the-Sea, north of San Francisco. Although every step of the run here would be familiar, running a marathon every day wouldn't be. This first state would be our shakedown cruise, our time for settling into routines that would carry us across the USA.

Between April 21 and May 1, George Billingsley and I would pass through Sacramento, the largest city on the transcontinental route... we'd join up with running friends in the Slice 100-K race... we'd climb from sea level to the High Sierra in our 260 California miles.

**DAY ONE.** Word had leaked out that we were attempting the run, and two newspaper reporters wanted to do a preview story. I refused, telling them, "We're merely running with our mouths at this point." Now we were ready to run with our feet.

But running was still incidental today. This first day was ceremonial—planned partly to allow time for the drive from home to the start area, but mainly so that two of my children and their spouses could see us start and bid us "bon voyage."

We chose Jenner as the starting point because it had not been associated with any transcon run. We wanted ours to be distinctive.

My younger daughter, Susan, and her husband, Ed Granlund, took camcorder shots of the start and along the way. My son Mark, a good distance runner as well as a published author, could not run with us because of an Achilles tendon injury. He had to settle for taking still photos.

Mark's wife Sabine, an excellent ultrarunner, did run with us. Well, to be honest she ran two miles with us, then decided the pace was too slow and scooted away.

Any athlete who has experienced the anticipation and anxiety of a contest of consequence knows the relief that comes once the event is underway. All our planning was now becoming operative.

The five miles of running were effortless and pleasant, even though road conditions were unfriendly to running. We hoped the narrow, curvy highway with poor shoulder conditions and heavy traffic wasn't a preview of too many days to come.

When we finished at Casini Campground, where we're spending the night, Susan and Ed surprised us by breaking out champagne and hors d'oeuvres. We drank to the success of the adventure we'd named "RUNXUSA."

Tonight, before launching this journal, I re-read the notes scribbled earlier about runs across the USA. I knew this was a massive undertaking, but considering that I was pacing to finish in 125 to 130 days (about 25 miles daily), I felt my effort was pantywaist compared to what the fast transcontinental runners and walkers had done.

As far back as 1909, Edward Payson Weston—at age 70—walked from New York to San Francisco 37 miles a day. The following year, he walked from Los Angeles to New York at a 46-mile-a-day clip. Weston was a professional walker who'd become wealthy from the sport.

Don Shepherd, a 48-year-old South African, claimed a transcon record in 1964 when he ran from Los Angeles to New York (3200 miles) in 73 days and eight hours. Reading in the *Guinness Book of World Records* of this performance, Bruce Tulloh of England thought it was soft and decided in 1969 to better it. He did by crossing from L.A. to New York (2876 miles) in 64 days, 21 hours.

True, Tulloh did make a faster journey. But my sentiments were still with Shepherd because he ran 324 miles more, was

15 years older, and had no support crew, whereas Tulloh had people following him in three different vehicles.

Frank Giannino of New York reportedly set the current record in 1980 by racing across the USA in 46 days, eight hours (San Francisco to New York City, 3100 miles). Giannino's performance was so astounding, however, that many ultrarunning experts question its validity.

The note that really made me feel like a running marshmallow was this: "Mavis Hutchinson at age 53 ran across the USA in 69 days. She is from South Africa and has seven grandchildren."

What's more, I even knew about a guy named John Enright who had gone across the country in a wheelchair. But the ultimate was Bob Wieland, who, in Vietnam, had lost both legs just below the torso. While sitting on his butt and using his arm strength, he'd pushed himself across the USA.

Well, I thought, at least if I do make it to the Atlantic, I'll be the oldest person to ever walk or run across the USA. Turtle pace be damned!

As I finished reading the notes, Elaine was just finishing the after-dinner cleanup. She had this satisfied look on her face, and I knew why. She had prepared a tasty dinner and had succeeded in getting me to devour all 5000 calories of it.

She has firmly resolved to stoke me with calories every day to minimize my weight loss. I had told her, "Shepherd lost 33 pounds on his run and Tulloh, six."

The gauntlet was tossed and she picked it up with fervor: I will lose less than Tulloh.

Thinking of Tulloh again made me conscious of how relatively few training miles I've put in. While preparing for his run, Tulloh logged 150 miles a week. My weekly mileage since last October has averaged only 73.

My original plan was to train 25 to 26 miles several days in a row to test my reactions to this distance that will now be my daily target. I didn't get beyond 15 miles.

Frankly, I now think I'm lucky not to have tried the longer runs. They might have discouraged me from starting what begins for real tomorrow morning.

**DAY TWO.** George Billingsley and I first met a dozen years ago when we crossed paths while training for the Western States 100-Mile Endurance Run. We became regular training partners, getting together at least twice a week.

Although he's only a kid of 68, George and I come from similar backgrounds. He had a military career, with the Air Force in his case, then had a second career, as an economist with the state of California.

Like me, he's now retired and has an undying fascination with long-distance running. I'm thrilled that he decided to come along on RUNXUSA.

As George and I started at seven o'clock this morning, we were both anxious to see how we would feel after our first 26-mile day. We'd agreed to make 10- to 20-minute pit stops every five miles to down some sort of snack.

Running through the Russian River resort area stirred memories of my high school days when I used to spend three weeks each summer at a Christian Brothers' camp located between Monte Rio and Moscow. I remember the crazy swimming meets we had in this river. One event was an underwater swim. I usually won because I had a better sense of direction than Evan Jenkins, who could stay under twice as long but couldn't travel a straight line.

Another event was the high jump (for form, yet!) from a tree perch 30 or 35 feet high. Jim Conway and I alternated as winners because we were the only two guys wild enough to make this jump.

Then there were the five-mile hikes to a picnic and swim area. Miles Cosgrove and I always ran the distance, and he was always too fast for me to catch. Miles, like Olympic runner Glenn Cunningham from the 1930s, had had his legs badly burned in his youth.

At camp, we took long swims in the river. My personal record was five miles. That was almost 60 years ago, so my interest in endurance tests isn't new.

During today's run, I was relieved to find that my three most vital pieces of running gear worked well: shoes, sacroiliac belt and fanny pack.

The New Balance 840 shoes proved to be comfortable and stable. Since I am running across the United States, I want shoes made in this country. New Balance meet that requirement.

I've worn a sacroiliac belt the past 10 years while running and racing, but it has been a small belt—only six inches wide. Anticipating added back strain on RUNXUSA, I opted for a bigger, stronger belt. The one I bought (for a whopping $163!) is nine inches in width—quite a load for an ancient and skinny runner, especially when it's soaked with sweat.

The belt compensates for a back condition with a tongue-wrenching name, "spondylolysis." This is a stress fracture in the arch of the vertebral bone that makes up the spine.

The fanny pack was a gift from Dr. Ralph Paffenbarger, with whom I've run more than 1000 miles side by side in races. The pack has three pockets, each zippered, and to that I added a pouch to carry a water bottle.

The pockets carry such items as a Swiss Army knife, a canister of mace (a gift from Doyle Harris after I'd been bitten four times by dogs), a $5 bill, a handkerchief, toilet tissue, suntan lotion, mosquito repellent and sometimes a snack. The belt and the fanny pack total about six pounds. Considering that race horses are handicapped with 15 pounds, this is not a light load to carry across the country.

The water bottle holds only eight ounces, just enough to get me from one pit stop to the next. It has to be light and soft enough to bang against me without hurting. I blush to confess that my choice is a baby bottle.

**DAY THREE.** George was in unusually high spirits today. In fact, we both were after starting the day feeling no undue strain from yesterday's 26 miles.

George spent today spouting the lines that have long made him an ideal running companion. He's a talker, and his talk is usually upbeat.

When we came to hills, he said, "I love hills." If there were a mosquito attack, "I love mosquitoes." While we ran in rain, he said repeatedly, "I love rain."

In at least one respect, George is a dyed-in-the-wool redneck. He wouldn't be caught in a restaurant, or most other public places, without his ball cap.

"This is probably the main reason why I haven't run the Comrades Marathon," he said of the world-famous 90-kilometer race in South Africa. "If I went there, the urge to ride the Blue Train would be overwhelming. But they would not allow me to wear my ball cap in the dining car. So, rather than suffer the disappointment of not riding the Blue Train, I haven't gone to South Africa."

Going through Calistoga today revived lots of memories for me. Back in my high school days on hunting trips with Bert Fitzpatrick, we would invariably stop at the Calistoga Creamery for giant-sized milkshakes that cost a quarter. The creamery, which has long since met its demise, never let us down for quantity or quality.

Another memory loomed as I saw Mount Helena. Elaine and I once jogged the road up the mountain on a hot day. The views of the Napa Valley and its vineyards were spectacular that day. But we had made the ascent without water and were parched on reaching the summit. A ranger mercifully supplied us with drinks.

Later in today's run, George and I reached the Silverado Trail where most of the Napa Valley Marathon now travels. I harbor fond memories of Napa for three reasons: the years I spent at a Christian Brothers' high school in the Napa foothills; this town was the scene of my fastest marathon, 2:39:38 at age 54; and this is the home of Jonesey's, where Elaine and I have enjoyed many a delicious and romantic dinner.

George and I ran at a slow pace all day and felt fine when we finished. We're spending the night in pleasant and familiar surroundings at Boethe State Park near Saint Helena. It's here where I do the day's writing, which is hereby done.

**DAY FOUR.** I don't yet feel that we have gotten into the run. Maybe this is because it has all been well-known territory to me so far. It will remain so until we leave Carson City, Nevada—which makes me anxious to get to that point.

For want of entertainment, I indulged in some mental gymnastics with George as we ran. The subject of Shakespeare came up. I mentioned some of his sonnets, and tried to explain to George what a sonnet and iambic pentameter are. I met with little success. The moral here is you cannot lead a redneck out of the pasture of prose.

Today, my left knee and a bone in my left foot both announced some discomfort. I reduced the "static" from the foot by putting moleskin on the sore spot and covering the moleskin with Elastoplast tape—both of which provided padding.

But the knee is a different matter. All of this January, I couldn't run because of an injury to this knee. My orthopedist ran a series of tests (X-ray, bone scan and MRI) but could not diagnose the problem.

During the month the knee was injured, I tried all kinds of devices to run on it. None worked. So I'm worried now because, if that knee goes whacky, I know of no remedial action.

After finishing our daily stint, we drove a short distance to Solano County Park for an RV hookup. The setting on Lake Solano is pleasant, but the toilets and showers are almost unusable. The buildings are also marred with graffiti, documentary evidence of the "sickies" in our society.

**DAY FIVE.** George was especially talkative today. He spent considerable time relating his experiences while working for the state of California, and educating me on the technicalities of appraising real estate.

He also entertained me with his Army experience in Panama, pre-World War II, when he enlisted as an 18-year-old. The most ribald of these tales is best not repeated here.

I related to George what I'd read about the Bunion Derbies. These were coast-to-coast footraces in 1928 and '29, organized by Charles C. ("Cash and Carry") Pyle. The races were conducted under rules that Pyle concocted, mainly to make money. For example, he routed the race only through cities that paid for the privilege. The race was computed by totaling the time it took each runner to cover the daily distances.

The 1928 Bunion Derby covered 3422 miles from Los Angeles to New York. Of the 275 starters, 55 finished. Winner Andy Payne, a 19-year-old part-Cherokee from Oklahoma, took 573 hours and collected $25,000 in prize money. George said, "That amount of money sounds paltry." But I pointed out, "In those days, it was enough for Payne to pay off the mortgage on his dad's ranch and to have cash left over."

In 1929, the race was run in the opposite direction—New York to L.A. Though the course was 200 miles longer than the year before, winner John Salo beat Payne's time by 48 hours while edging Englishman Peter Gavuzzi by a mere three minutes. Nineteen of the 91 starters finished.

I reminded George that, in these two races alone, 74 people had run across the country. Then I added, "Technically, these guys did not run entirely from coast to coast contiguously, because they crossed the Hudson River and the Mississippi River by ferry." Our plans call for crossing rivers only by bridge. Hey, this contiguous thing is important to us!

The routine for our day is evolving. We're up at 5:30 a.m. and start running by seven. We run for about seven hours but are on the road an hour longer because of our pit stops every five miles.

After we finish running, the routine is: grocery shop, find an RV park, shower. Elaine prepares dinner while I work on my log.

Then we do our other homework: check navigation for the next day, check for RV parks near our finish, lay out gear. Our luxury is to read a daily newspaper or some book before falling asleep early.

**DAY SIX.** Today's run was unique in that George and I did not have the frequent pit stop services of our wives. We spent most of the day on Sacramento's American River Bike Trail where there either was nowhere to stop or no paralleling road for vehicles.

While running on the bike trail, our RUNXUSA T-shirts drew attention. A few bicyclists and walkers asked, "What do those letters stand for?" Others wanted to know, "Are you really running across the country?"

We met my daughter-in-law Sabine on the bike path as she was out for a 25-mile ride. Sabine has a good understanding of what George and I are attempting.

A native of West Germany, she has finished the famous 100-kilometer Biel race in Switzerland that attracts nearly 25,000 competitors. She also has won the women's division of the Lake Tahoe 72-mile run.

We had a pleasant visit but cut it short a bit so we wouldn't miss our rendezvous with Elaine and Georgia in Goethe Park. As Sabine biked speedily away, George and I both wished we were endowed with some of that 26-year-old energy.

Every so often running along the trail, I saw a mile marker that remains painted on the pavement from the Carson City to Sacramento 166-mile races of 1984 and '85. Run at the rate of 41-1/2 miles per day over four days, it was my longest race ever. That experience has given me a certain amount of confidence for RUNXUSA.

Several times today, George and I expressed surprise that, after five days, of running we're not more tired or sore. The day wasn't without problems, however.

Estimating that we had a mile or two yet to run, we passed by Elaine and Georgia who yelled and waved to us from a pathway near the bike trail. We returned the greeting and kept going. We were actually only 500 yards from the finish in Goethe Park. But we failed to recognize it and ran on past.

Two miles later, a bicyclist dispatched by Elaine caught up

with us to report our mistake. We were pooped after running back to the ladies.

They asked us in no uncertain terms, "How could you be so infernally stupid?" Like chastened puppies, we bowed our heads in shame.

**DAY SEVEN.** We ran less than our average today because we'll do 62.2 miles the next two days. This weekend is the Slice 100-kilometer race, run at 50-K (31.1 miles) per day. Along with Ray Mahannah and Hal Stainbrook, I have directed this event for nine years. The course varies every year, but it is always in some part of the Gold Country.

I have run all these races with Ralph Paffenbarger, a world-renowned epidemiologist from Stanford University. We wanted to keep the string going to qualify for the 1000-kilometer award by finishing 10 races. It soon became evident to me while planning RUNXUSA that the only way I could run the Slice 100-K this year would be to make it part of our cross-country route.

I queried some of the entrants about this idea, because it would require them to climb from 250 feet elevation to 5000 in the Sierras. They wholeheartedly endorsed it as a send-off for George and me.

Being a part of the race this weekend complicated our routing today. We had finished about five miles from the Slice start yesterday and didn't want to run so little today, nor did we want to duplicate any of the race course.

Thus, the only way we could extend today's mileage was to drive to the Slice finish line in Hams Station and run 13 miles from there, then return to Sacramento to complete the linkup with the race course. After running in the scenic high country, we found the remaining miles through the city rather blah.

Elaine and I met Dr. Ralph Paffenbarger soon after he checked into the motel. "Paff" told us that he has suddenly found himself with a big problem. "I'm not too sure that I will be able to get through this year's race," he said.

That very morning, in a routine physical exam, a cardiologist had discovered heart-muscle damage in three areas. Paff made reference to "silent ischemia," and I'm not sure exactly what this means except that it has something to do with decreased blood supply.

"One of the strange things here," he continued, "is that the cardiologist is unable to tell me how the damage occurred. The reasons he can't are that I have no record of previous symptoms, and this is a new setting—the first time he has examined me."

After a pause in which Elaine and I tried to absorb all this, Paff said, "My cardiologist would strongly disapprove of my being here for this race."

I was torn between shock, concern, and disbelief. I've run with this guy for years, and he's a virtual animal. Still vivid in my mind is the time when I paced him for part of the Western States 100-Mile Endurance Run. We were going down a rough, rocky trail, and he was flying.

"My God," I thought then, "this guy is running 100 miles and I'm running only this 10-mile leg with him. I'm busting my ass to keep in contact with him so he will have access to the water I'm carrying. He's running effortlessly and smoothly, and I'm struggling."

And this guy has heart trouble?

I finally asked Paff, "What do you intend to do about the problem?"

He replied, "The cardiologist recommends a four-way bypass. But before submitting to that, I will try to correct the problem by modifying my lifestyle—better diet, more sleep, reducing the workload." Knowing his zeal and enthusiasm, I doubt if he will ever keep the resolution on workload.

Tonight, Elaine, Paff, and I went to an Italian restaurant so we runners could load up on carbohydrates. We were joined by my elder daughter Nancy and her husband Dan Phillips, and by my son Mark and his wife Sabine.

It was a cheerful gathering, but I found myself harboring much concern about Paff. I realize that if this could happen to Paff—a considerably tougher and more enduring runner than I—it happen to me.

I had always thought that, after I died, they would have to take my heart out and beat it to death with a baseball bat. Now I am not so sure.

**DAY EIGHT.** When Paff told me last night that his cardiologist would not approve of his being in this race, he also said, "I will make a concession to that doctor. I will take it very easy in the race. You can run ahead if you want."

I told Paff, "No way. We've already run eight Slice 100-K races together, visiting and enjoying. I am not about to scoot away and leave you."

In fact, with nearly 3000 miles to go after the Slice race, I welcomed a slow pace today. Paff, George, and I started an hour ahead of the other runners to keep us from unduly delaying the finish. Besides, it gave us a chance to say "hello" as they passed us.

As we started, I felt somewhat guilty about leaving Hal Stainbrook and Ray Mahannah, my co-directors for this race, with all the responsibility. Hal handled all the pre-race chores, and Ray did the marking of the course and the timing.

We agreed that Paff would set our pace, which seemed the best way to stay within his limits. He hit upon an easy-to-handle mix of jogging and walking.

About the time that we got to the mounds of rocks left over from the gold-rush days, runners began to catch us. Leading the way was Dave Stevenson.

Funny how some memories linger, but I always associate Dave with the delicious cookies his wife treated us to during the 166-mile run. Jeopardizing his lead, he took time out today to slow down and chat before wishing us good luck and speeding away.

Jerry Blinn, Roland Martin, and Steve Galvan ran together as they came upon us. Jerry reminded Paff, "This is my eighth Slice, and I'm only one behind you."

Roland, who's built more like a fullback than a runner, said he had no doubts that George and I would finish RUNXUSA. Steve, who races almost every weekend, cautioned us to pace ourselves across the country.

It was more fun when the women came along. All but one of them stopped to hug me. The fact that all these young, pretty women—Toni Belaustegui, Joan Bumpus, Linda Elam, Joann Hull, Dee McKim and Sharlene Kelley—would stop in the middle of a race to hug a sweaty old man shows the high respect they have for a guy running across the USA. My God, think of the scenario if I were a handsome young stud!

The one woman who didn't give me a hug was Pam Martin, a newcomer to the race who didn't know me. She did stop long enough to wish us luck, then went on to win the race. The moral here is, if you want to be a winner, don't stop to hug sweaty old men.

Seriously, I will carry the warmth and good wishes of all these runners with me all through RUNXUSA. I appreciate their gestures of friendship in coming to this race to wish us well.

Even with the slow pace, all three of us were tired when we

finished. This makes us fearful of tomorrow when we will gain over 4000 feet in elevation in the 31.1 miles.

Paff, Elaine, and I are staying overnight at the new Shenandoah Inn in Plymouth, along with Ray Mahannah. We ate dinner in nearby Sutter Creek at Belotti's Italian Restaurant, an eatery that holds fond memories for Elaine and me from our courting days.

**DAY NINE.** We started even earlier today, 90 minutes ahead of the other Slice 100-K runners, and walked more than yesterday. The milder effort agreed with me, as I felt surprisingly strong all day.

Like yesterday, but unlike all our other days on the road, we did not make extended pit stops at five-mile intervals. Instead, we simply exchanged greetings with Elaine, grabbed our food and drink, and kept going.

During the entire 31 miles, Paff, George, and I kept up a steady stream of conversation. Paff told a memorable story about running the Comrades Marathon in South Africa last year.

In this case, "marathon," is misleading because the race is not 26.2 miles. It varies in length from 54 to 56 miles, usually the latter nowadays.

Comrades, the world's most famous ultradistance race, dates from shortly after World War I. It began as a memorial to soldiers in that war.

Paff bubbled with enthusiasm in talking about the race. "In 25 years of running," he said, "I have never seen such a well-organized event."

Amazingly, it has 13,000 starters, and more than 10,500 of them finish. Paff told of his excitement on running into the stadium at the finish to the cheers of 30,000 spectators. Every bit as encouraging, he recalled, was that along the entire route fans stood to see the race and yell encouragement to the runners.

"There's one thing about this race that many people in our country don't recognize or understand," Paff told us. "It's free of any racial overtones or discrimination. Black runners are as welcome as white runners, and they are all treated equally."

He added, "There's one catch to Comrades. There is an 11-hour cutoff time. They enforce it by locking the doors to the stadium so that any runner who can't finish under 11 hours is not admitted."

I wondered if, at my age, I could make it before the door slammed in my face. We do know now that we can make two 31-mile days in a row while climbing high into the mountains.

Now it's back to our daily 26-mile average. Piece of cake!

**DAY TEN.** Today we fought the fury of the mountains and tasted their majesty. Until now, we had been running in T-shirts and shorts. But we started this morning bundled in polypropylene tops and tights, covered with Goretex jackets and pants.

The temperature was 22 degrees, and a strong wind made it feel much colder. The severe wind persisted all day, gusting to 50 miles per hour at times.

In the miles approaching 8573-foot Carson Pass, we encountered heavy rainfall and were apprehensive that it might turn to snow. This would have made the going dangerous, if not impassable, for the motor homes. We couldn't allow them to become stranded on the mountain.

George and I had barely reached the summit before light snow began falling. We told Georgia and Elaine, "Drive down from the summit as fast as you can safely go. We'll catch up with you below the snow line, no matter how far away that is."

For George and me, going down the mountain was every bit as taxing as going up. Because of the wind and slippery highway, we had trouble keeping our feet under us. When a car approached, we had to plant ourselves and not move to keep from sliding into its path. Luckily, few cars were on the road.

This was undoubtedly our toughest day to date. But despite these difficulties, the beauty of the area wasn't lost on us. El Dorado Forest, Silver Lake, and Caples Lake—no matter how many times seen—are always inspiring.

What impresses me most about the area is its ruggedness— the mountains of granite rock. In history books, I've seen pictures of pioneers working their way through this region, and now I marvel even more at their feat.

On a paved highway and moving only ourselves, George and I still had a rough time. I feel like a prima donna compared to those pioneers.

I also feel a little like a pioneer in another sense. After taking leave yesterday of Mark and Sabine, I realized it would be more than four months before I'd see any members of my family again.

I had previous experience being separated from family, on Marine Corps duty. When Mark and Nancy were youngsters, and Susan was not yet born, I'd done 14 months' duty in Japan while they remained in California.

But now I have Elaine here with me, and thank God for that. I thought, during today's toughest miles, how comforting it would be to reach the coziness and warmth of the motor home, and roost for the night.

Despite the weather problems, I am on easy street as far as food is concerned. Elaine is getting into her program of keeping me well-stoked on pit stops and at dinner.

The girl is determined that I will not lose weight, and so far she's succeeding. I weigh exactly the same as when I started nine days ago. To Elaine, that is victory.

# E S S A Y

## *The Shuffler*
### by Bill Glackin

*(I first stood in awe of Bill when we were seniors in high school. In academic competition with hundreds of other students in California, he ranked first to win a four-year college scholarship. Bill has for more than 40 years been a highly respected arts reviewer for the Sacramento Bee. In 1980, he was a runner-up for the Pulitzer Prize for criticism. In 1984, he was chosen for a Conservator of American Arts Award—becoming the first critic so honored. — Paul Reese.)*

Paul Reese was always a Doer. I mean, whatever there was to do, he got it done faster and in better shape than anybody might reasonably expect.

One of the earlier examples I recall was the fact that he got his master's degree (in political science) from the University of California at Berkeley in two semesters and a summer session instead of the usual two or even three years. As a fellow grad student bumbling along at an even slower rate than the norm, I was deeply impressed.

But not surprised. We knew each other well by that time, having met in our freshman year at Christian Brothers High School in Sacramento. The friendship we formed quickly has lasted more than 60 years so far, despite the fact that life has often put a lot of distance between us.

We did our undergraduate college work separated by the Berkeley hills, but managed to spend a lot of weekend and summer time together.

Those were the swinging years in popular music. The Benny Goodman Band was leading the way, often on bandstands in northern California, and the determination that was part of Paul Reese the Doer popped up in an odd place, the dance floor. While maintaining with steadfast modesty, or perhaps realism, that he had "no sense of time and two left feet," he pursued the music of the great bands in the company of some pretty and truly charming young women—not one of whom ever complained, in my presence at any rate, of getting stepped on.

His idols were, oddly enough, not the most famous swing leaders. He preferred such individualistic personalities as Cab Calloway and Phil Harris, who sometimes took time off from the Jack Benny radio show to lead a very good band through the ballroom circuit.

World War II separated us again—he was in the South Pacific, I in the Aleutians. But we kept in touch, and I wasn't surprised when he wrote to me that, after dangerous times reconnoitering the Solomons in the dead of night, he had finally achieved what had been his original ambition in the Marines—to get into the air. The Doer had done it again. (He subsequently flew 96 missions.)

As much as any of this, though, it was a note from him while he was stationed postwar in Japan that left me flabbergasted. As a flatland golfer and tennis player with a low level of ambition, I was in awe of somebody who could run up to the top of Mount Fuji and back just for the fun of it.

Which brings us to Paul Reese the Runner, and his marvelous, inspiring achievement in running across the country. Marvelous and inspiring, I might add, regardless of age.

When he told me he was going to do it, I could hardly believe it. When he did it, I was stunned. This was surely the greatest "Do" of them all.

Then I finally put two Do's together. (This is called making a two-Do out of something.) Just before Paul and Elaine moved to their present home, they lived for a time not far from our house, and I would see Paul running on the neighborhood streets.

It was my first glimpse of the running style I think of as

the "Hundred-Mile Shuffle." It seemed to me that his feet hardly left the ground.

Thinking of Paul doing that across 3000 miles of America, I suddenly made a connection to that long-ago shuffle on the dance floors of Rainbow Gardens in Sacramento and the Coconut Grove Ballroom in Santa Cruz. Do you suppose that's where it all started?

# Overview of Nevada

**May 1 to May 17, 1990 — 405.2 miles — 655.5 total**

| Day | Overnight | Miles | Notes |
|-----|-----------|-------|-------|
| 11 | Minden | 25.1 | last 11.9 miles in Nevada, temperature 27 degrees |
| 12 | nr. Carson City | 25.0 | George injured |
| 13 | Fallon | 25.4 | first taste of desert |
| 14 | Fallon | 25.5 | |
| 15 | east of Fallon | 25.0 | temperature hit 106 degrees |
| 16 | w. of Frenchman | 25.3 | adopted earlier starting time |
| 17 | w. of Cold Spr. | 25.0 | temperature dipped to 25 |
| 18 | west of Austin | 26.1 | temperature 20 |
| 19 | east of Austin | 25.4 | temperatures 10 to 91! |
| 20 | east of Eureka | 25.1 | completed 500 miles, temp. 29 |
| 21 | near Eureka | 26.0 | |
| 22 | east of Eureka | 26.0 | temperature 25 |
| 23 | west of Ely | 26.0 | temperature 22 |
| 24 | Ely | 25.0 | |
| 25 | Majors Place | 26.2 | temperature 26 |
| 26 | w. of Baker Jct | 26.2 | temperature 19 |

(first 10.5 miles in Utah on Day 27)

## Chapter 2

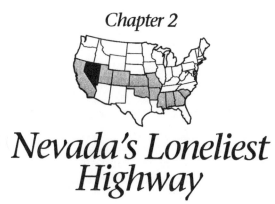

# Nevada's Loneliest Highway

Exiting Carson City to the east, we entered new territory. Every mile run from here to the Atlantic would be new.

We knew that the Nevada desert would be dry and empty. But our research also revealed the surprising facts that we would cross eight mountain passes of 6000 feet or higher, and we might encounter some of the COLDEST weather of the trip, as well as the hottest.

George Billingsley entered the new state with an injury troubling him. I wondered, as we faced 405 miles between May 1 and May 17, "Could I be next?"

**DAY 11.** Today held two highlights—one running, one personal. The day was a running milestone in that we put California behind us. This brought feelings of progress but also a feeling of cutting strings to home.

The personal highlight: This is Elaine's and my wedding anniversary.

George was troubled all day with shinsplints. "I have no idea what caused them and little idea of how to get rid of them," he said. I was of little help to him on that score.

To try to get his mind off his injury, I peppered him with idle conversation. He showed the most interest when I reported the advice that Annabel Marsh had written in a letter when she learned of our transcon attempt.

Annabel, at 61, is the oldest woman to run across the USA. She was accompanied by Caroline Merrill, a mere child of 42 years. Annabel had advised us, "Use motels rather than camp out. You will need a shower and a good bed at the end of each day."

George and I agreed that a shower is a genuine treat after

running all day. But we also decided that traveling by motor home is more convenient—and cheaper—than relying on motels.

Annabel had also said, "You will need a big bucket or pan to soak your feet every night in ice water." I have the bucket but haven't used it yet. George has been icing a knee and soaking his feet, and he says that Annabel was on target with this suggestion.

I am following one piece of Annabel's advice literally: "Be sure to eat a lot on the way." Elaine and I estimate that I'm stoking in at least 7500 calories a day. Here, George lags quite a bit behind me.

Annabel had said that she and Caroline started out eating quite nutritiously, but after several weeks they devoured everything in sight and still lost weight. I told George that Annabel's total weight loss was 10 pounds.

Knowing George's passion for McDonald's caramel sundaes, I recalled Annabel saying she and Caroline thrived on hot fudge sundaes. They formed an attachment to Dairy Queens, which often were the only places open at night in small towns.

I never got around to clarifying another of Annabel's suggestions. She'd suggested that our pit crew stop every 2-1/2 to five miles so we could get water. This gave the impression that she and Caroline didn't carry water.

George and I each wear a fanny pack and drink every 20 minutes or so. George is much better disciplined about this than I am. He drinks heartily while I sip only an ounce or two.

Maybe Annabel hadn't carried water because her approach to a running day was different from ours. She and Caroline would have a very light pre-run snack and then take off for 15 miles of running. They would then stop for breakfast and rest, and run another 15 miles in the afternoon.

They also would take off every Friday. Their six days of 30 miles had totaled 180 a week. Our 26 miles every day added up to 182-mile weeks.

Before starting, George and I had talked about various approaches to the running day: 26 miles continuously, 13 in the morning and 13 in the afternoon, or splitting the day into three runs. We agreed to stick with the continuous 26 miles and to try another approach only if we ran into trouble.

I couldn't help but chuckle when I recalled one of Annabel's suggestions. She'd said, "Bring along a good book to put yourself to sleep at night."

George almost went into hysterics when he heard that one. After a day's run, sleep comes almost as quickly as turning off a light switch.

I remember clearly an oddity of Annabel's and Caroline's trek. They had gone through 27 pairs of running shoes between them in their 3200 miles.

By that standard, I was going to come up a half-dozen pairs short. George and I had figured on seven or eight pairs each.

When we finished running today in Genoa, Nevada, Elaine gave me a bad time because I'd promised there would be a grocery store here. Not so. The highlight of Genoa was a spot claiming to be "the oldest bar in Nevada."

We had to drive to Minden for our grocery shopping. While Elaine shopped, I hurried off in search of anniversary flowers.

I found a florist and bought a dozen carnations. Elaine then outdid herself in preparing an elegant dinner. One thing's for sure: we'll never have another anniversary like this one.

**DAY 12.** When the Billingsleys arrived at today's starting line in Genoa, I jumped out of our motor home, ready to run. George came over and said, "We've got to talk."

"Sure," I told him, "we can talk as we run along."

"No, you don't get it," said George. "This is important. We've got to talk NOW."

At that, all sorts of thoughts raced through my mind. Did George have a major problem with our modus operandum? Had he decided this is not for him and he is going to quit?

In short order, George related that his shinsplints had him in deep trouble. He could barely walk. He said, "I've given it some serious thought, and I want Elaine and you to go on ahead. I'll try to catch up in a few days if I can."

He would push on as best as he could by just walking. He made it emphatically clear that he didn't want me going along with him.

I told him, "My viewpoint is that Marines do not leave their wounded on the battlefield. Somehow I am going to keep tabs on you."

When I talked this over with Elaine, she agreed. George and I would stay in some sort of contact unless he decided to quit the expedition altogether.

George would have no part of me walking with him, so I would run three miles ahead, join Elaine in the motor home and wait for George to arrive. Once he showed up, we would know he was okay and I'd shove off on another three-mile leg.

This became the routine for our day. Every time I saw George come in, he clearly was hurting. He remained grittily determined, though, to log at least 25 miles for the day—no matter how long it took. Seeing him in this condition, I found myself feeling somewhat guilty because I was running so injury-free.

Near Carson City, I felt good enough for some playing around. I hopped off the road and ran a hundred yards on the actual Pony Express Trail, treading in the footsteps of history. Though it has been more than 40 years since I read a book about the Pony Express, I still remember one fact about it: The riders could not weigh over 120 pounds.

Once we left Carson City on Highway 50, I entered territory I'd never run before. This added an air of excitement to the excursion.

But whatever elation I might feel is now tempered by concern over George's problem. He felt justly proud of himself for making today's 25 miles. But we face tomorrow with all sorts of questions weighing on us.

**DAY 13.** The shinsplint injury again limited George to walking—and painfully at that—so we followed the same procedure as yesterday. I ran three miles ahead, visited with Elaine, and enjoyed grub and grog until George showed up.

I checked on his condition, then ran three more miles. George is firmly resolved to put in a minimum of 25 miles a day, and he has the bulldog tenacity to hang in until he accomplishes that mission.

Near Dayton, I saw signs marking the Pony Express Trail. I concluded from studying the scene that there could have been much trouble from Indians in this area because any rider could have been seen for miles. There is no place to hide. Once again, I relived a part of history by running a few yards on the Pony Express Trail.

I stopped later to talk with two bicyclists who were on a cross-country tour. They said they had started in New York, and I expected to hear that San Francisco was their destination. Instead, they told me, "We're headed for the Humboldt Redwoods in far-northern California."

I admire these guys for being entirely self-sufficient. They carry their own sleeping bags and pads, cooking and eating gear, clothes, toilet articles, and a few quart bottles of water each. One of them said, "We bike from 60 to 100 miles each day, depending on the terrain, the weather, and our mood."

I hadn't realized as we left the Dayton area that we would be cut off from civilization so abruptly. Dayton itself has a surprising amount of buildup, and I noted that new homes can be purchased for $58,000. That price tag and the proximity to Carson City are probably the attractions.

Once out of Dayton, though, we passed quickly into the desert. About the only signs of civilization are the highway, the fences, and some telephone poles.

But I ran so easily in the mild weather that I kept asking myself, "Will the desert continue to be this kind?" I had anticipated miserable heat, dryness, and dehydration.

I marveled at the pioneers who had crossed the desert. For me, it's a breeze with food and drink awaiting me every three miles, and shelter if I need it. For them, it was an endless struggle—not enough water, too much heat, equipment breakdowns, limited food supply.

Even such a simple act as going to the bathroom (to put it euphemistically) was complicated for them. How did they ever do that with a semblance of privacy in these wide-open spaces?

Through the barren desert, Elaine and I anticipated civilization when we arrived at Silver Springs. Instead, we found the town consisted of a mini-market, a post office, a small cafe, and a few homes.

A sign outside the cafe read, "Coffee 5 cents." I wondered if that was true, or was it a sign left over from the good old days?

The height of sophistication at Silver Springs was a truck watering the dirt roads. As we left town, a sign told us that cattle could be on the road for the next 17 miles. Ah, companionship at last!

We finished our day 23 miles west of Fallon but decided to drive there for a couple of reasons: we needed to stock up on groceries and propane, and we wanted an RV park and hookups. Tonight's warm, soothing shower was pure luxury.

**DAY 14.** I am beginning to realize that my favorite part of the day is early morning. There seems to be a cleanliness about it, and the quiet beauty of a dawn unfolding is never tiring. There is no hurly-burly, and Elaine and I seem to pretty much have the world to ourselves for a few moments.

At 6:30 this morning the sun shone brightly on the desert

highway. Seeing the farmers in their fields and the city workers scurrying to their jobs, I felt lucky that Elaine and I can take a slice out of our lives for this experience. We are blessed.

For seven miles this morning, I was king of the frontage road paralleling Highway 50. I didn't meet a single car.

But a new problem arose as mosquitoes dive-bombed me. They resurrected memories of Guadalcanal, only thankfully these buzzers are not anopheles—a "tribe" whose name I'd probably not be able to spell except that I remember it well from having had malaria three times in the Solomon Islands.

At one point, two dogs ran out barking and looking threatening. Recalling lessons learned from a dog book (*Dog Watching* by Desmond Morris) that my daughter Susan had given me to prepare for the day when Elaine would get her dog, I exuded friendliness. Or at least I made a gallant effort to do so.

Surprisingly, the tactic worked. I won over the dogs to the point where they ran along with me for a half-mile, often getting between my legs and almost tripping me.

After the barrenness of the desert, the approach to Fallon with the commercial strip on its outskirts came as a stark contrast. I thought at first that the strip signaled nearby city limits, but it started seven miles out of town. Fallon, with a population of slightly over 4000, looked metropolitan after a day in the desert.

Waiting for me in town, Elaine had visited with a glider pilot, Alex Burnett, and his wife who had given her a preview of the road ahead. They'd reported that we would cross at least eight summits of 6000 feet or more before leaving Nevada.

Alex had also warned, "Stay off the historic Highway 50 route because of the grades, curves and road conditions."

Today was kind of an even-keel day—no major ups or downs. But I thought several times of how, within the same day, covering the mileage can turn from a piece of cake to bread and water.

I did all my running solo because George is still ailing. He is mending slowly and remains as determined as ever to keep going. But I can see that he's tired, too. As evidence of that, his wife Georgia offered him a McDonald's hot caramel sundae at the 23-mile mark. He refused this treat, which he usually regards as an epicurean delight. This is like a lion refusing red meat!

**DAY 15.** An assessment process starts each day. I check my body for chinks in the armor. The two most frequent complainers are my left knee and left foot.

Over the past few days on the desert, I've acquired the first physical problem that is staying with me. This is the condition of my lips.

At first, they were just chapped and annoying. Now they are cut and bleeding, and eating or drinking anything hot is painful.

When running, I cover my mouth with a red bandanna, which was Elaine's idea and a good one. Now I understand why the cowboys wear those bandannas.

I met up today with two women bicyclists on their way to New York. They estimated they'd arrive there in two months.

A support vehicle carried all their belongings, plus an extra bike and parts. A smart approach, but softer than the one taken by the self-sufficient bicylists we'd met two days ago.

I envy the bicyclists for their ability to cover mileage so fast. On the other hand, I prefer the freedom of my feet over the rigidity of a bike. If I were to spend a day hunched over handlebars, even a chiropractor would not be able to straighten me up.

Today, I also encountered two long-horned cows with three calves. At first, I worried about those longhorns and their protective mothers. But the cows turned out to be more fearful than I. Confused, they ran down the side of the road ahead of me for two miles before heading out into the desert.

We played a bit of fool-around while passing a cathouse east of Fallon. We'd been told that it had been doing a prosperous business until the commanding officer of the Fallon Naval Air Station put it off-limits to service personnel. Killjoy!

At any rate, the establishment still stands with all its signs and decor. Elaine and I have the camcorder scenes to prove it.

With George still battling his injury, I had a lot of time for thinking—and maybe a little hallucinating. The mountains to the east seemed to get farther away all the time, though I was supposed to be gaining on them.

Then I thought: How many people can say, I climbed Mount Everest, I was an Olympian, I was an All-American, I swam the English Channel, I ran across the USA?

I will be in somewhat elite company if I accomplish this. But "elite" only by the sheer quantity of the feat and not by the quality of my performance. After all, a 53-year-old grandmother and a walker have done it faster than I will.

Even at my pace, there is a price to pay for all this. Nonetheless, for me the price is right—a bargain, in fact.

Elaine and I are having a ball. Making the transition from the comforts of a three-bedroom home to a 20-foot motor home takes some attitude adjustment, but we are managing well.

Would that everything in life were as simple and well-defined as what we are doing now. Run 25 to 27 miles, and the day is a success.

As we go along, Elaine and I are developing a fascination with the desert. I am becoming aware of how much stillness there is out here, and the fact that the desert wind is an almost constant companion.

**DAY 16.** Elaine and I added a new feature to our day. We were on the road at 5:30 a.m. This by a guy who, before starting on this trek, had vowed not to be on the road before seven o'clock. But with the heat mounting, I considered the 5:30 a.m. start a stroke of genius.

After finishing in 106-degree weather yesterday, I wondered if the temperature would go higher today. (It didn't. The high was a mere 90 degrees.)

Of more serious and immediate concern was the danger of getting hit by a car. I am learning that running on the left side of the road, facing traffic, isn't safe. A car going the same direction as I am and passing another car going that way can come dangerously close to me. I do not see it coming. There's just a frightening "swoosh" sound as the passing car roars by. Then I get an aftershock effect and feel the wind the car creates.

Ninety percent of the motorists I encountered this Sunday morning were inconsiderate, forcing me to the dirt shoulder. By contrast, the majority of truck drivers moved over to give me running room.

Unlikely as it seemed out on this barren desert highway, a sign read, "Low-flying aircraft next 1/4 mile." Then another sign told me that I was adjacent to the weaponry target range of the Naval Air Station. I hoped those guys were accurate.

Near Fairview, I stopped to read a historic marker of the Tonopah-Goldsmith silver boom. The town had 27 buildings—including bars, hotels, saloons, a miners' union hall and a newspaper—in 1906. Two years later, the boom had passed and the townspeople fled after mining $3.8 million worth of silver.

Another marker told about the Wonder Mine, which

produced $6 million in gold, silver, and copper between 1906 and 1912. What impressed me most was that this community had its own ice plant and swimming pool. Talk about fringe benefits!

Most of the route today was through rolling hills, the road bordered with green sagebrush and wild grass that extends to the foothills. As I came to each crest, the question was, "What's on the other side?" The answer was always: "More of the same."

Remote from any RV park or motel, we're spending the second night in a row camped at a safe spot off the highway. The main problem with this arrangement is our limited water. Our motor home water tank holds only 36 gallons. To be on the safe—and comfortable—side, we carry another 12 gallons in two-gallon bottles. But with drinking, cooking, bathing, and toilet flushing to do, the water supply still requires constant monitoring on the desert. By comparison, 300 to 500 gallons a day for a house is not unusual.

**DAY 17.** If my memory serves me correctly—which it doesn't always do these days—it was King Richard who said, "My kingdom for a horse!" These nights as I go about writing this log, I can paraphrase that as, "My kingdom for a typewriter!"

We did not bring a typewriter because of our limited space, and not since World War II have I been so long separated from one. Quite often each night, as I write longhand in the log, I have to stop and rub the cramps out of my writing hand. Maybe the fact that it is swollen from the heat has something to do with that.

George has perked up a bit, and we ran 18 miles together today. He told me, "I've already cooked up three projects to be undertaken on my return home: build a cat walk attached to the back of our house to give Georgia's indoor cats an exercise area, trim the eucalyptus trees near the house, and cut away some of the brush intruding upon our 300-foot driveway."

I wondered what brought on this rash of creativity but restrained myself from commenting. He also reported, "After 350 miles of travel, the cats are now adjusted to life on the road. They now stare out of the motor home windows like tourists."

A sign along the way told us that we were again beside the Pony Express Trail. Since George had not read much about the Pony Express, I shared a few salient facts: that the riders carried pistols but not rifles; that they earned $30 a month; that Buffalo Bill Cody was a rider.

In turn, as we saw some cows, George contributed to my bovine education. "Dairy cattle, such as Jerseys and Holsteins, are more dangerous and meaner than beef steers," he said. He also told me that a cow with a new calf will defend it to the death and that if you are searching for a cow that's just given birth, she is easy to find because she emits a delicate "moo."

At my first pit stop, I saw that Elaine had taken on a new project. She's making a pair of infant pajamas, departing for now from her crocheting and guitar practicing. She tried to instruct me, unsuccessfully, in the art of making buttonholes for the pajamas.

At the next pit stop, Elaine greeted me with warm vanilla pudding over bananas as part of her continuing campaign to keep my weight up. So far, I've lost only one pound.

At day's end, when I removed my shoes in the motor home, Elaine commented, "Those shoes smell like gas. Anything that smells that bad has to be deadly."

I took a whiff and admitted to myself that they were, indeed, ripe. So much so that I agreed with Elaine's suggestion and hung these dear companions outside to air until we go to bed. I'll bring them in for the night because they might attract some hungry coyote!

**DAY 18.** The temperature at our 5:15 a.m. start stood at 19 degrees. With the windchill factor, even with my sheepskin gloves I couldn't keep my fingers warm. At this early hour, we owned Highway 50, which a roadside sign called, "The Loneliest Highway in America."

I did the first 20 miles with George—slowly because he is still battling injuries, but gamely so. Our talk turned to how the pioneers got water while traveling through this area. This prompted George to recall his experiences of building a home in Alaska while stationed there on Air Force duty.

"In Anchorage," he said, "pipes were laid three or four feet deep in gravel in some areas. In other areas, the muddy ones, the water pipes went 15 feet down. In Fairbanks, with permafrost, the depth was two feet."

Later, George told me a story about a horse named Kitty. When he was in the seventh grade and living in Oregon, a nearby dude ranch let kids take a horse home for the winter— a good deal for the ranch, which got free board and room for the horse, and a good deal for the kid, who owned a horse for the winter.

"Kitty had a broken jaw as a result of an accident," George told me, "and this jaw never set properly, so Kitty's tongue was forever hanging three or four inches out of her mouth. I rode Kitty to school each day, 3-1/2 miles one way, and stabled her there with other horses when I was in school. The kids with horses had a club of sorts, and we ate our lunches in the stable."

Kitty, overworked on the dude ranch, was obstinate at first. But after George fed and pampered her for a while, they bonded. He said that was a winter he hated to see end. The parting was hard for both Kitty and him.

The scenery is changing. A small pine tree, the first I'd seen for endless miles, signaled the shift. Clumps of junipers then appeared every so often.

Coming through New Pass Summit, I got a view that looked like the Swiss Alps. Mount Airy Summit brought an equally spectacular sight before we descended into a valley and encountered range cattle on the road.

A jackrabbit scooted across the highway and in another half-mile we came upon a rabbit that had not made it across. Every game has its winners and losers.

Coming down from Mount Airy, Highway 50 leads to Austin in a straight line for eight or so miles. I hurried those last miles so that Elaine and I could be tourists in Austin, a colorful mountain hamlet.

While Elaine was busy in the town's laundromat, I walked the length of town—five blocks or so—camcording interesting scenes. I was told that the International Hotel and Cafe here were moved piece by piece from Virginia City, and that the town once had its own 2.8-mile railway.

After finishing the laundry, Elaine did some grocery shopping. I tried my luck on a slot machine and won $5.

Our chores completed, we then drove back west along our route to rendezvous with George and Georgia, and to camp at Reese River Valley. We couldn't pass up the chance to stay at a spot so appropriately named.

**DAY 19.** Reese is a big name in these parts, but that's not all good. I had read that the Reese River Navigation Company, operative during the mining heydays, bilked some Eastern

investors out of money. The pitch was that money would be
made from shipping ore on barges down the Reese River. Turned
out the river was only inches deep, which the Eastern investors
learned the hard way.

Back to reality at the 5:30 a.m. start in 10-degree weather.
My hands were miserably cold, even though I was wearing
heavy sheepskin gloves, until the sun popped over the hill an
hour later.

The cold weather does help to earmark potential injuries.
I'm finding, for example, that the annoying bone in my left
foot hurts more in the cold. George says his shin splints also
bother him more in this weather.

I remarked to George this morning, "Our endeavor should
make us eligible for purple hearts." This prompted George, an
Air Force veteran, to relate a war experience.

"I was on an LST in World War II when it was sunk," he
recalled. "Many survivors were picked up by a destroyer, and
all those with any wounds were taken to sick bay. Everyone
sent there automatically got a purple heart—including the guys
who burned their hands going down the escape rope and one
who somehow cut himself while evacuating ship."

I countered George's report by telling him the story of a
Marine in World War II who was guarding a Japanese prisoner.
"The prisoner bit him and, as a result, the Marine was given a
purple heart."

Then we got off on a discussion of whether the many airmen
who got purple hearts for frostbite deserved them any more
than the service personnel who contracted malaria. For sure,
both were much more deserving than rope-burn awards.

When we reached Austin after about six miles on the road,
I felt as if I were visiting an old friend—after spending a pleasant
afternoon here yesterday. The town now has a population of
400 or so, but at the height of the mining boom it was home
to 10,000.

Running into the town today, I got a good view of Stokes
Castle. Built by Anson Stokes, a rich Easterner who had extensive
mining interests in the area, the castle can be seen for miles.

It is a replica of a Roman tower, three or four stories in
height and made of hand-hewn granite slabs. No one lives in
it now.

Just before we entered the town, we passed a man sleeping
on the roadside in his sleeping bag. His shoes rested near his
head, and his jeep stood nearby. Seeing him like that made us

happy for the warmth and comfort of our motor homes.

Going by Kent's Grocery, I was reminded of the honesty of the folks in Austin. Yesterday, after I had won some money in their slot machine, the proprietor came out from behind the counter to make sure that the machine had paid in full. It hadn't, so he pushed a second button to give me all I had coming.

I reminded myself to tell people that Austin, Nevada, is a town with personality. They should meet her someday.

Austin's postmaster told me that the winter temperature here sometimes goes as low as minus-10 degrees. The elevation is about 6800 feet, and today we climbed nearby passes as high as 7600 feet.

The first 17 or 18 miles consisted entirely of going up or down. It was exciting to have something new unfold around each turn, rather than more of the same desert ahead for 20 miles or so.

It was also refreshing, after the flat desert valleys, to pick up the pace running down the hills. But I flirted with danger here—the danger of overdoing it, running too fast and injuring my quads.

The route flattened and straightened out again for the last eight miles. One advantage of such roads is that I can see approaching cars. Another is that finding parking spots for pit stops is easier for Elaine.

When I come into the motor home where Elaine is stopped, I play a guessing game on the mileage covered. Too often, the tripometer reads less than I had hoped to see.

At one of my late pit stops today, I announced to Elaine that tonight I would remove the Elastoplast that has been wrapped around my metatarsals for three or four days.

She replied, "What toxic waste dump is it going to?" No respect.

**DAY 20.** I began the day with a feeling of achievement, knowing that we would pass 500 miles. We're getting someplace, I thought, but this elation was offset by the realization that we still have more than 2500 miles to go.

George attempted to stay cheerful this morning despite his ongoing battle with shinsplints. Only 10 miles out, George was already hallucinating. He said, "I hope that when we reach Eureka there will be a McDonald's." He made plans to indulge in a hot caramel sundae with nuts. His morale dropped a notch later in the day when he discovered that McDonald's has not invaded Eureka.

While traveling alone I found the day somewhat dull, so I amused myself with a game. During walking breaks, I'd close my eyes and see how many steps I could take along the highway's white fog line without straying from it. My record was 51.

Obviously, this also required some intent listening for oncoming cars. But Highway 50 is so lonely that seeing a car is more unusual than not seeing one. In this setting, with the road endlessly the same (an impression intensified by being afoot and moving so slowly compared to vehicular traffic), the miles stacked up very slowly.

Today, to relieve some of the strain on my left leg, I ran 10 to 12 miles with—instead of against—the traffic. A bit scary.

Years ago, while foolishly running with traffic in a three-day race, I'd been hit by a big, black Cadillac. Luckily, no serious damage was done.

Drivers were more curious than dangerous today. A gent in his mid-50s, bearded, looking like an outdoor type, stopped his battered green coupe, adorned with the words "Spirit Wolf." He asked, "Are you going across the United States, too?"

His question caught me off guard at first. How did he know? Then I realized he had talked with George, who was trailing me. I nodded yes.

"Are you doing the run with only that gear?" he asked, pointing to my fanny pack. I told him about having a motor home for support.

Later, a Cadillac stopped and the driver yelled, "Hey, wanna ride?" I hollered back, "No, thanks." I felt more like shouting, "Let's hear it for the good Samaritans!"

At my last pit stop of the day, I changed clothes since the weather was warming. To do this, I had to take off my shoes.

As their aroma filled the motor home, Elaine commented, "I'd rather walk through fresh cow patties barefoot than step into those shoes!"

True, the shoes are a bit ripe. But they've carried me 500 miles without injury—without even a blister—and I'm sticking with them.

**DAY 21.** It wasn't a relaxing night. A violent storm hit as we camped in a nondescript roadside area. The gusty, whistling winds were eerie and scary as they swayed the motor home.

We placed all our luggage and equipment on the floor for ballast. And still the motor home, which we'd pointed into the wind, rocked ominously. This wasn't a night made for sleep.

Going by a ranch this morning, George and I saw 12 bulls—many of the Brahman breed. Some had mean-looking horns and, I suspected, as they glared at my red outfit, accompanying mean dispositions.

Confirmed farmer that he is, George was fascinated by the cattle and with studying the barbed-wire fences. He gave a discourse on the art of stretching barbed wire, but I didn't listen very intently. Barbed wire simply doesn't do it for me.

George mentioned how he is looking forward to running through his birthplace of Hardy, Arkansas. I responded with an Arkansas story.

"When I reported for Marine Corps officer training in Quantico, Virginia, I was immediately impressed with my company commander, First Lieutenant Sidney McMath. In speech, appearance, and action, he was 100-percent officer-like. McMath looked like a young George Bush, and he let it be known that someday he hoped to become governor of his home state of Arkansas. After the war, he was elected to that office.

"But I read in the national press that tragedy struck during his administration. His wife shot his father when his father tried to force himself upon her, and McMath went no further in politics."

At the next pit stop, George exited his motor home before I left mine. Elaine and I looked out and burst into laughter as we saw George walking down the highway—in the wrong direction.

I tooted vigorously on the motor home horn and got him turned around. Now I had ammunition to heckle him for a while.

I began by telling him, "The word 'retreat'—as you were doing—is not in the Marine Corps' vocabulary. Marines may 'tactically withdraw'—but retreat, never!"

George returned to his farmer mode as a cow with a calf—which George estimated to be one week old—ran fearfully away from us.

George explained, "When a cow has a calf, she likes to get off by herself with the calf because this hastens and strengthens the bonding process. A calf born among a herd of cows often has trouble in identifying its mother, and the bonding process is complicated."

Watching George plunge ahead, day after painful day, I hope that if an injury comes down upon me, I will be as stoic as he in maintaining our 25- to 26-mile-per-day average.

As we approached the town of Eureka, I felt like a pioneer coming off the prairie into the protection of a fort. We would find an RV park with all the luxuries (water, electricity, and sewer hookup) in Eureka, if we were lucky.

Like Austin, Eureka is located in a pass. But the cut here is nowhere as dramatic as the earlier one was. The town sign reads, "You are entering the loneliest town on the loneliest road in America."

Our dream of a luxurious night didn't come true. The town's RV park left so much to be desired that we're again camped at a roadside rest area.

**DAY 22.** The best part of our running day is the early hours when we "own" this small area of the earth and witness the dawn unfolding. In the first 2-1/2 hours on the road this morning, George and I saw only eight cars.

I am also beginning to conclude that the toughest miles each day—those that add up the slowest—come between 11 and 17. They aren't the most difficult physically, but psychologically.

I tend to recoup as the end of the day's running draws nearer. Why this is the pattern, I'm not sure.

Saddened to come in for a pit stop and to hear from Elaine that the radio reports Sammy Davis, Jr. is on his deathbed. As a college student 50 years ago, I first saw him perform with his father and uncle at the Golden Gate Theater in San Francisco. Then, about five years ago, Elaine and I saw him at Lake Tahoe. A great evening in which, to everyone's delight, he sang "Candy Man" and "Bojangles."

Hey, thanks for all the pleasant memories, Sammy—and God bless! Out on this lonely road, I am saying a prayer for you.

While running, I make it standard operating procedure to wave to every motorist who moves over for me. This adds up to a lot of waving in one day, yet I get satisfaction from this split-second rapport.

Not all encounters on the road are satisfying, however. Today, a black Chrysler driven by a well-coiffed woman of about 50 (and smoking, I noticed) bore down upon me and chased me off the shoulder.

"What the hell was that all about?" I wondered. Not wanting to waste any energy at this stage of the day, I restrained myself from giving her an obscene gesture.

And, let's face it, she was probably so fascinated with my legs that she lost track of where she was going. You know, pilots sometimes get target fixations. She had legs fixation!

Running along, I spotted a black mustang who was watching me. He began to play games. When I ran, he ran. When I stopped, he stopped.

I yelled to him, "I see you out there, partner. You're beautiful!"

This referred as much to his being the embodiment of a free spirit as as it did to his physical appearance. Almost as if he understood me, he ran a small circle to show off. Then he ran away from me. To freedom.

Watching him move so rapidly, I silently thanked him for the entertainment.

**DAY 23.** George reported today that the pain from his shinsplints is waning. But now his knee, on which he had arthroscopic surgery three years ago, is beginning to give him trouble.

At our first pit stop, George said he would delay there to doctor his ailing knee. As I pushed on alone this early morning, the only noise in the desert was the sound of my feet hitting the pavement.

While looking up at sandstone cliffs six or so yards from the highway, I almost expected to see an Indian standing atop them. Why is it in these early hours, as I go through the desert and see no wildlife, that I have the feeling that dozens of eyes are upon me?

Up popped a thought about the kid who worked at the service station in Austin and who said he was going into the Marine Corps in a couple of weeks. After seeing my license-plate frame for the motor home that reads, "Alumni, USMC," he'd asked me for some advice about the Corps.

I gave him a few suggestions. Later, I regretted not giving him 10 minutes of instruction on close-order drill. How I would have liked to have had it in 1941 when I reported into Quantico, Virginia, for officer training.

I still recall a gang of us officer candidates getting off the train at Quantico. A sergeant there to meet us yelled, "Fall in, dress right, right face." I didn't have a clue what he wanted us to do.

For the first time in 560 miles, I dropped my water bottle today while drinking on the run. Only some quick footwork kept it from rolling off the highway into a deep gully.

I'd learned this fancy footwork while working as a busboy in college. In those days, when I dropped a dish, the trick was to break its fall with my foot so the dish would hit the floor with little impact and not break.

Elaine's ingenuity and imagination always add a lot to my day. Practically every time I come into the motor home for a pit stop, she has dreamed up a different kind of treat.

One of these days I will have to catalog all her different culinary offerings. This morning it's banana nut bread.

I can never outguess her on what the treat will be. Yesterday, for example, it was sumptuous lemon loaf breakfast cake.

The importance of having Elaine sharing this trip with me and caring for me cannot be overstated. If I make it across the country, as much credit belongs to Elaine as to me.

Damn, what do I mean IF? WHEN I make it across!

Oh yes, it's Mother's Day. I'd remembered it was coming and bought Elaine a small memento, a musical heart, when in Eureka. It's handcrafted needlework with an implanted musical tune, "You Light Up My Life." To get the song to play, you push a little button in the back of the heart. It's supposed to last for 10,000 repetitions. I should live so long!

At one pit stop today, Elaine said, "All I want out of life at this moment is a garbage can and a mailbox." We're getting to the basics.

**DAY 24.** George must be feeling good because he began the day with some banter, saying, "Maybe I will loan you one of our cats." That's humor, because he knows the last thing in the world I want is a cat.

Don't get me wrong—I don't have anything against cats. It's just that I am violently allergic to them.

As mentioned earlier, one of the conditions that George's wife Georgia set in agreeing to the trip was that she take her three cats along. Hell, George was so eager to run across the USA that he would have agreed to taking along a gorilla.

This morning, we started where the foothills touch the desert valley, working our way upward through several passes that snake through the mountains to the summit. I fought the mountain by running most of it. As a result, I'm somewhat tired tonight—but better off than the many dead jackrabbits I saw along the road today.

I pushed the pace to hasten our arrival in Ely so Elaine could get the burglar alarm on the RV repaired, stock up on groceries, get gas, do laundry, and take care of a number of other tasks. That surge of energy surprised me. Sure would like to patent it.

On the downside, a bone in my left foot gave me trouble today, and I have a new theory about it. It's most likely arthritis. It hurts sometimes when I'm lying in bed. If it were an injury, it should hurt only when bearing weight.

Unusual procedure today in that I cut the umbilical cord about two-thirds of the way along and asked Elaine to drive on into Ely to transact her business. Armed with a peanut butter and jelly sandwich, a Mars bar and a bottle of water, I set off solo after her departure.

Unluckily for me, rain began to fall a short while later. It was a long haul into town solo, but it increased my appreciation for Elaine's pit-crewing.

When I found her in Ely, she was bubbling with enthusiasm over the service a mechanic there had given her. "I told Bill Sanford about the run and the fact that we didn't have time to wait around," she said. "He dropped everything and repaired the burglar alarm on the motor home and aligned the front wheels."

Tonight, to celebrate the rejuvenation of the motor home, we followed Bill's suggestion and had dinner at the Jailhouse Restaurant.

This might be Ely, Nevada—population 4882—but the food, service, and setting would rival any metropolitan restaurant. Hey, much more of this and we'll be too soft to hit the highway again and take off toward the Atlantic Ocean!

You know, I suddenly realize I'm enjoying this experience more than our recent cruise to the Panama Canal—which is saying quite a bit. I guess the reason may be that you enjoy the do-it-yourself experiences more. Here, Elaine and I are doing rather than just viewing.

**DAY 25.** Shortly after starting this morning, George found a weather-beaten penny. He figured this would bring him good luck.

I told him, "We've already been lucky with the weather. Bill

Sanford, the Ely mechanic who worked on our motor home, told us he has seen Fourth of July parades canceled here because of snow."

George's penny must have worked. He reported later that his knee was improving.

As for me, though, a sharp, jolting pain unexpectedly radiated up my left thigh today. It happened three times, almost like an electric shock.

I need to monitor that and put some Aspercreme on it. Aspercreme, moleskin, and Elastoplast tape are my angels of mercy.

I spent my whole day facing traffic, with my left leg down. In order to stay off the corrugated bike path, I have to be on the highway itself.

The only safe way to do that is to be facing traffic. Were I to go with traffic, I could wind up a statistic—like all those KIC (killed in crossing) jackrabbits.

I encountered a live jackrabbit, and he ran parallel to me before disappearing into the sagebrush. I clapped my hands to try to make him jump (amusement is not easy to come by out here!), but he didn't take the bait. Smart rabbit.

Somewhere around 500 miles, Elaine and I discovered that we were riding a high wave of confidence. We had no doubt about continuing at this 25- to 26-mile-a-day clip.

Putting in the mileage has sort of become like going to work each day and getting the job done. Getting sidelined with an injury or getting hit by some careless driver are the two major concerns.

I've taken to wearing a watch on each wrist. The one on the right wrist is for time of day. The one on the left wrist is a stopwatch which records the actual time on the road between pit stops.

Three observations from the road today:

1. Most of the local pickup trucks whizzing by are equipped with all-weather tires that emanate an irksome whining sound.

2. Sheriffs' cars and Ely police cars are constantly in sight, patrolling. Does this indicate a high crime rate?

3. As I passed a historical marker, some tourists drove to the roadside sign. They stayed in their car to read it instead of getting out for a short walk. That is Americana 1990.

**DAY 26.** At breakfast, Elaine said, "When I looked outside last night, there were so many stars that it looked like the sky had measles."

This was our last full day in Nevada, and we would pass into Mountain Time Zone (an hour later than Pacific) at the Utah border. George and I discussed a plan to adjust to the new time. We would start 15 minutes earlier every two days until we'd made up that hour.

Today featured my run-ins with snakes. Early in the day, I almost stepped on a four-foot snake coiled and slumbering on the highway to warm itself.

At our last pit stop, we came across two snakes. Later I was going down the road alone when a lizard crossed the road and zipped between my feet. Had he been a sidewinder, I would have been in Utah in five minutes.

Two motorists stopped to talk with us, one right after the other. A guy from Colorado parked his car and joined us for a half-mile, briefing us on what to expect in his home state.

He left, and shortly after a Nevada Highway Patrolman (only the second we'd seen since leaving Carson City) pulled alongside for a chat with us. It was evident that his bottom line, though unspoken, was to verify that we had vehicular support.

We thought it fitting that we should cross Sacramento Pass, which shares the name of the major city nearest to our hometowns. The ascent to the 7174-foot summit was deceiving. It looked easy at first but developed into a tough pull.

The approach was different from the other climbs. They had gone through narrow and curvy passes, whereas here the passes were mostly straight and wide. This would be the last summit we had to cross in Nevada.

At today's finish, the four of us held a powwow on a plan to see the Lehman Caves in the Great Basin National Park, America's newest (established 1986), sometime tomorrow.

We decided on our usual 5:30 a.m. start and on running without a pit stop until 7:30 a.m. or so. Then we will mark the spot where we stopped on Highway 50 and go back for the 9:00 a.m. tour of the caves.

At Baker, we will also take on gas and groceries because the next provision place is Delta, Utah, 100 miles to the east. More importantly, we will fill up with water. Our main logistical problem on the desert has been maintaining an adequate water supply.

We're camped tonight beside the highway. Oh well, the price is right.

# E  S  S  A  Y

# *The Needler*
by Pete League

*(Pete ran his first road race in 1951 at age 14. During the 1960s, he competed with mixed success in the Philadelphia and San Francisco areas. He has been founder/promoter/race director of numerous events in California, Texas and Ohio. Pete continues to run. — Paul Reese.)*

As I enter my fifth decade of involvement with running, three people (aside from my late father, Eddie League) immediately come to mind as examples of role models for excellence in athletics, family life, and friendship: Browning Ross, Bob Carman and Paul Reese.

Paul and I met in 1965. I was working in Sacramento, and Paul had recently retired from the U.S. Marine Corps and taken a job in Sacramento as an administrator with the city's secondary schools.

We struck up a conversation prior to the annual Lodi-to-Stockton 15-mile run. This was clearly a day one would like to remember: 90 degrees at the five p.m. start, and no water stations on the course that I can recall.

We often speak of that race because it was the first for Paul and his son, Mark. It was also one of my better attempts.

Our relationship was nurtured through many training runs in and around the Sacramento area, and the occasional race during the late 1960s. I recall one of Paul's early marathons was Las Vegas in 1967. He won his division, and Mark set a national age-15 mark of 2:45:18. Pretty impressive stuff back then!

Paul believes in "putting back what one takes out," and he soon became involved in organizing races. By then, I had put on a number of events myself.

One day, Paul came to me and said, "Pete, we need a

good, tough ('tough' is a word one uses when thinking of Paul) 20-mile race here in Sacramento. We (as in 'you and me, Peter!') should do it."

The Pepsi 20-miler was born. Having grown up with a running background in the Northeast where road race awards are often merchandise (first person in gets first pick, etc.), Paul and I went door to door and came up with all manner of awards. The race was immediately the most popular one around—a far cry from those giving 39-cent medals and plastic trophies.

I left Sacramento in late 1967, but the friendship has endured. A trip to Paul's area is incomplete without a phone call or dinner, and the letters from him have continued.

The man stays up nights thinking of ways to needle me in one manner or another (all in obvious good humor). Also, no matter where I travel, I bump into this guy. At London-to-Brighton, there's Paul; at Boston, there's Paul; at the Dipsea race, there's Paul. Always with a friendly needle and open arms.

When I read Paul's original journal of his run across America, the story that struck me most and is typical Reese was his comment when his original running partner, George Billingsley, developed shinsplints and told Paul to go on without him.

He said, "We Marines don't leave our wounded on the battlefield!" Then he kept tabs on George for a week or so while his injured partner had to walk to recover.

# *Overview of Utah*

## May 17 to May 30, 1990 — 338.5 miles — 1003.0 total

| Day | Overnight | Miles | Notes |
|-----|-----------|-------|-------|
| 27 | nr. Utah border | 25.0 | last 14.5 miles in Utah |
| 28 | west of Delta | 26.5 | |
| 29 | west of Delta | 26.2 | |
| 30 | Delta | 25.5 | |
| 31 | near Holden | 25.1 | RUNXUSA one month old |
| 32 | Salina | 25.0 | |
| 33 | east of Salina | 25.0 | |
| 34 | near Emery | 26.0 | winds 35 to 40 MPH |
| 35 | w. of Green Rv. | 25.0 | temperature 29 degrees |
| 36 | w. of Green Rv. | 30.5 | |
| 37 | Green River | 25.0 | |
| 38 | e. of Green Rv. | 25.1 | George found $135 |
| 39 | near Cisco | 26.5 | ran in first heavy rain |

(first 11.1 miles in Utah on Day 40)

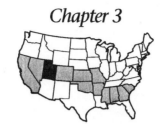

## Chapter 3

# *High and Dry in Utah*

Utah promised to be as high and dry as Nevada, but with more scenic delights as compensation. We also looked forward to reaching two milestones: completing the first month on the road early in this new state and passing 1000 miles just before leaving Utah.

However, we brought a new concern into this state. Could we run these 338 miles without interruption? At times, we had no choice but to use the freeways. While it is legal to run on Interstates in Utah (unlike in most other states), I could not locate the letter I had received from the state's highway department that confirmed this.

Would the highway patrol try to stop us? We'd test the tolerance of these officers between May 17 and May 30.

**DAY 27.** There was a feeling of achievement as we exited Nevada and entered Utah this morning. But this was one of those days when my brain wasn't fully in gear, because we were four miles into the new state before I became aware that every mile of the highway is marked with a green sign. I could now watch the miles add up.

We interrupted our running to drive to Great Basin National Park and to tour the Lehman Caves. We were told these are among the largest limestone solution caverns in the Western USA and contain many stalactites and stalagmites.

"Both grow at the rate of an inch each century," the guide said. "These formations have been millions of years in the making."

Reflecting on all the history here makes a person with a life span of 70 to 80 years feel fleetingly transient. Comparatively, a human lifetime is like a drop of water in the ocean.

Because we lost so much time with the four hours out for the Lehman Caves excursion and driving time, plus the hour time-zone change, I shortened the pit stops today. Made 'em gulp-and-go.

Didn't see a single building on Highway 50 once we left Baker Junction. I thought, "If this road were a corporation, it would be out of business." Fifteen or 20 minutes sometimes passed today without my seeing a car.

A man I judged to be about 60 stopped his pickup and told me that he had a message from George. He was trailing me today as he again humored an injury. The driver chuckled and said, "George says to slow down."

We talked briefly about the beauty and fascination of the desert. Before driving off, he said, "I sure take my hat off to you two guys."

Oh, the thoughts that go through a man's head. Over the past few days, I've observed that about 35 percent of the vehicles on this road are RVs. Ninety-nine percent of them are driven by senior citizens.

I reflected on our likable mechanic in Ely and remembered the last thing I saw him do as we left: take a snuff box out of his pocket and put a pinch against his gum. I wanted to say, "Hey, knock that off because it's likely to lead to cancer and loss of your gums and jawbone." Instead, I remained politely silent. Did I do the right thing?

At the end of our 25 miles, we reached the base of the foothills and decided to roost here for the night. When we embarked on this expedition, I had concerns about mountains. Now I welcome them as relief from the desert valleys.

Troubled off and on all day with some sort of twitch in my left knee. At one point, shooting pains almost buckled the leg.

I suspect that the shoes I'm wearing are about at the end of their usefulness after 680 miles of RUNXUSA plus 70 training miles. They're going into retirement and on to the Great Stinky Shoe Heaven. Faithful soles they've been.

I wind up the day with some thank-you memos on my mind: Thanks for no rain, thanks for the wind which reduces the heat, thanks for my faithful New Balance 840 shoes to which, on the occasion of their retirement, I dedicate this day.

**DAY 28.** The new pair of New Balance 840s I broke out this morning helped to absorb the shock of the hard hit on the chipped-gravel pavement. I realized right away that I'd worn the last pair of shoes much too long.

If I want the shoes to absorb the shock, I've got to reduce the mileage on them. Five hundred miles is the limit.

As I've said before, it's nice to be running across the USA in a pair of shoes made in the USA. With all the nice things I've said about New Balance without an endorsement, imagine what I'd say with one!

Oh joyous day, I ran down that steep descent without any injury indication whatsoever. Hallelujah! I always like these descents when I'm injury-free. They seem sort of like a free ride.

Much as I enjoyed the downhill today, George took the opposite view. His gimpy knee rebelled when he ran downhill.

While we ran together, George reported on the farmer who'd stopped to talk to us yesterday. This was the fellow who had relayed the message from George to slow down. "We talked at the Nevada border where he was waiting to sell some alfalfa seeds," said George. "He has a 1200-acre spread in Utah which he works with two of his sons. His other two sons went to college and never returned to the farm."

George was impressed with the man's ties to earth and his fondness for farming.

After George and I parted company, jackrabbits kept me entertained. One jumped out near me, and I tested my new theory about stopping rabbits.

I chanted to him in a singsong tone and, presto, he stopped dead still to listen. Then as he moved off, I renewed the chanting and he stopped again.

What is this fatal fascination I have with rabbits? Am I on the verge of a great discovery?

Out jumped another jackrabbit. "Hi, there, Jacque!" I yelled. I tried my singsong chant on him. But he just ran away, completely ignoring me. I've never seen a rabbit run a straight line for such a distance. He needs to be sent back to boot camp for escape-and-evasion training!

Insects were also my companions today. The last 100 miles, I've seen many grasshoppers unfold brilliant orange wings as they fly. I also ran into some nasty flies with a bite that stingeth. The fun barometer dropped a bit as I fought them off.

No complaints, though. The cars could outnumber the flies, and that would be worse.

My allergies began to sprout, with the sinuses misbehaving and bleeding. If this persists tomorrow, I'll take an allergy pill—much as I dislike taking any type of medication when all's going so well.

We finished the day atop a mountain, a spectacular setting for our overnight campsite. Oh, luxury, it even has a garbage can!

**DAY 29.** The most difficult act each day is to roust out of bed at 4:30 a.m. But it is certainly worth the effort to enjoy the magnificent morning.

Elaine and I launched the running at 5:20 a.m. It was still dark at that hour, so I ran by her headlights.

After she broke away, I ran by flashlight to make sure the highway was snake-free. Highway 50 belonged to me as I ran down the center line. Out here alone, against the vastness of the desert, the mountain ranges and the clouded sky above, I felt Lilliputian.

George took a later start to adjust to Mountain Time. Georgia passed me shortly after six o'clock to signal that George was on the road.

In one hour, only two other vehicles passed me. That's the traffic volume I like.

A thought: "Take away the highway, the telephone poles and the litter, and you would never know that man has passed through this area." The litter, unfortunately, is a telltale indicator of American civilization.

Judging from the many disposable diapers dumped (appropriate word) roadside, many motorists with small children must travel this road. Either that, or a few kids are on a heavy laxative diet!

Friendly drivers brightened my day twice. A young family— mother, father, three girls—in a station wagon stopped to ask the familiar question: "Do you want a ride?" I declined graciously and silently thought, "What trusting souls."

I was daydreaming when a car stopped just ahead of me, smack in the center of the highway. The driver was Irish, the same farmer who had stopped to visit earlier.

He announced, "I'll catch you in Hinkley tomorrow and give you some fresh asparagus." Considering the price of asparagus, that sounded like a good deal.

Today's scenery unfolded as I had pictured the desert—flat, sandy, sagebrushy, barren—except that I expected it to be 35 degrees or so hotter. I kept warm this early, windy morning by wearing a polypropylene top, a pair of tights, a lined windbreaker suit, a knit cap, and a pair of sheepskin-lined gloves. Much concession to old age here.

The white flag went up this morning, and I surrendered to an allergy pill. Almost immediately, it put my sinus miseries on hold.

Later in the day, I came to a small knoll and could see the highway stretching for endless miles. No doubt then that we would camp overnight on the desert floor.

At the 25-mile mark, I came across a dead snake, about four feet in length. Elaine told me that she had seen a number of motorists reverse course to study it. Which again proves that entertainment is hard to come by out here.

Our finish line was singularly unexciting, but the good news is that Elaine located an excellent overnight spot. "Excellent" in this case is defined as flat, sufficiently off the highway, and with a firm foundation not likely to bog us down in case of rain.

**DAY 30.** Winds raged to about 60 miles per hour overnight, and we were again concerned about the stability of the motor home. We pointed it into the wind and, for ballast, moved our gear and supplies from the cab overhang to the floor.

After about three hours, the wind finally subsided and we relaxed. When I looked out the window, I saw the stars more sharply defined than I've ever seen them. The desert should be a good classroom for astronomy.

Just as I learned to adjust in combat, we are learning to adjust on this expedition. Living in a 20-foot motor home, Elaine and I are blissfully adjusted to each other. If we weren't, it WOULD be combat!

We are adjusted to overnighting on the desert valley and to the water conservation required here. We are still adjusting to getting up at 4:30 a.m.

That's the price we pay for the enchantment of early morning on the desert. George is still sticking to his 6:15 departure as part of his adjusting to the new time zone.

Now 80 miles or so into Utah, we still haven't seen a Highway Patrol officer. Nor have we seen a commercial bus any place in Nevada or Utah.

I wonder if Greyhound covers this route when not on strike. If so, it could be a loser.

My human contacts today were of the familiar type. First, a bicyclist stopped to pump me for information about farms and water between here and Nevada. I told him, "Best as I can remember, the next water is at the border, 80 miles west."

"I have six quarts and believe I can make it," he said. We wished each other luck and went our separate ways.

Later, a Utah resident stopped to ask if I was in trouble.

Same answer as always. Come to think of it, out here on this highway—bedecked in baseball cap, T-shirt, half-tights and running shoes, and carrying a fanny pack, do I look like a guy in trouble?

Approaching Hinkley, I saw many fields under cultivation—a striking contrast to the desert barrenness. The town looked impoverished. Its only business was a gas station. The general store was out of business, and the section of town that borders Highway 50 stood in dire need of housecleaning.

A road sign told me that 110,000 Japanese were interned in nearby Topaz from 1942 to 1946. Elaine said the countryside around here reminded her of the Boise Valley in Idaho where she was raised.

On this Utah Sunday, the next town of Delta was buttoned down. We were lucky to find a gas station and grocery store open, but could locate no place to buy propane.

Delta gave us no choice of RV parks. It had only one, and it sat in the center of town. Can you believe its name? Kitten Klean.

**DAY 31.** A memorable day in one respect: It marks the completion of our first month on the road. By my calculation—always subject to correction—we have stayed two nights in motels, 10 in RV parks and 18 on the roadside.

Another impression of the day that lingers with me is seeing the mountain ranges silhouetted against the background of dawn. This scene reminds me of pictures in World War II taken by our submarines, pictures of islands that we would soon invade. I can never get over how war experiences, 47 to 49 years removed, sometimes feel as if they happened only yesterday.

We soon discovered that the area immediately east of Delta is barren desert with heavy sagebrush growth some three feet high. The only signs of civilization these first few miles were the highway, the telephone poles and a ranch fence. I even passed by some sand dunes today, the first I can recall.

Later this morning, a car zoomed close by. As I stepped off the highway to give him room, I barely missed stepping on a dozing snake. I didn't stop for any introductions or handshaking.

From the front lines of the highway battle zone, I am saddened to report that the jackrabbit casualties today were heavy. Six purple hearts posthumously.

By mid-morning, 20 or more motorists had moved over for me. I gratefully waved to each one.

At 18 miles came a change of pace from the desert. For several miles along the highway, the area was cultivated in alfalfa. This was a big-time operation. I watched one farmer driving a John Deere tractor and towing a Hesston baler. The bailer picked up the alfalfa, then processed it into bales that stacked on a trailing wagon.

The size of the irrigation equipment impressed me. I was fascinated by the rainbow produced by the combination of the watering and the desert setting. Elaine saw it, too, while driving, and jammed on her brakes and stopped in mid-road to camcord it.

Today was typical of how circuitous Highway 50 often is. Much of the time, it heads south instead of due east. There are no mountains to interfere with a direct route from Delta to Holden, and I'm sure that a straight shot would have saved me a great deal of running distance.

As compensation, however, the last 10 miles into Holden were a sheer delight. The highway was blacktop with four-foot shoulders—plenty of running space.

Holden, we were disappointed to find, offered only a small market, a couple of gas pumps, and a post office. Sy's Trailer Park rented overnight spaces in his cow pasture for $7. The cows and their patties were too thick. We declined and found a roadside spot in a hayfield.

**DAY 32.** We could have run smack into a roadblock or a disaster this morning. But a reconnaissance that Elaine and I made yesterday saved the day.

Just beyond Holden, Highway 50 dovetails with Interstate 15 all the way to our next destination, Scipio. This combination of 50/15 is a freeway loaded with fast-flowing traffic I had no desire to face.

Luckily, Elaine and I were able to trace the old Highway 50 which is now a frontage road (and didn't appear on our maps). About half the distance to Scipio was pavement, slowly deteriorating, and the other half was gravel. The road had one rather steeply graded hill, but Elaine and the trusty Mallard were able to negotiate it.

George again elected to start later. He ran the frontage road by himself and sent Georgia away to Scipio via the freeway because he questioned their Minnie Winnie's ability to travel the back roads.

It's unfortunate that, judging from the present state of maintenance, this stretch of old Highway 50 won't be around much longer. What a blissful run it was with nobody but

Elaine and me on the road for 12 miles. Without doubt, this was the most relaxed stretch of running since we left Jenner.

It was an unusual experience to be running along this gravel road, hearing the crunch of my feet on the gravel, and at the same time seeing the cars on I-15/Highway 50 roaring along at 65 to 75 miles per hour. The steady stream of cars was racing between Las Vegas and Salt Lake City. I saw more cars in two hours than I had the previous two weeks.

Scipio sits in a valley with a big mountain range as its backdrop. As I entered the town, the road was now paved and an old Highway 50 sign still stood. Were I not such a nice guy, I would have copped it as a souvenir.

I stopped to talk with an old gent (look who's talking!) about to pick up his mail at the tiny post office. He told me that Indians led by Black Hawk had once raided the valley to steal the pioneers' cattle.

He pointed to a pasture and said, "My grandfather and another pioneer were killed in a raid there."

The old gent also said that he had served with Patton's army in World War II. "In tanks?" I asked.

"No, heavy artillery," he replied. I noticed that he walked with a distinct limp and was left wondering if he had been wounded in the war, or if the injury were this farm- or age-related.

Scipio marked the end of the dream road. I-15 split off from Highway 50 here, and I was again heading east on 50.

The day's run finished, Elaine and I decided to drive into Salina to get propane and check into an RV park. This could be the last one until Green River, 125 miles from here.

We're holed up at the Butch Cassidy RV Park. Can't get much more colorful than that.

**DAY 33.** West of Salina, the mountain ranges on both sides of the road peter out and give way to a series of foothills before dropping—severely—into the town. Atop a mountain, looking down into Salina, I saw it sitting in a small valley encompassed by mountains. I was elated with the 10-mile drop into town and the ease with which I ran it.

Three circumstances bolster the economy of Salina: First, it is blessed with abundant water. Second, Highways 50, 70, 89 and 24 all run through it to funnel in tourist trade. Third, the nearest competing towns are Delta, 67 miles west, and Green River, 125 miles east.

Walking through Salina to take in the sights, I stopped at

Mom's cafe, which proclaimed itself "a landmark since 1929," and bought coffee to go. I later regretted passing up the fresh strawberry pie.

What unfolded beyond today's 15-mile point could have been a disaster. Highway 50 virtually disappeared. Its name became linked with Interstate 70.

I-70 is a high-speed freeway with two lanes on each side of a center divider. No signs prohibit pedestrians, but Elaine and I decided to retreat and confer with George and Georgia, who were three miles behind us.

We had two alternatives: follow I-70 or reroute and add 150 miles (six days) to our trip. We agreed to take a chance on the Interstate. "So far," I told the group, "we've not seen a highway patrolman in our whole time in Utah. Now we'll probably see a dozen."

I know that somewhere in my routing file I have a letter from the Utah Highway Department, saying it is okay to run on this part of I-70. The question is, did I bring the letter with me? Haven't been able to locate it yet.

We had reached the 22-mile mark on the freeway when I suggested to Elaine that we try the frontage road. According to a local farmer, it ran for another 25 miles. This turned out to be safer and more relaxing. But as we neared the end of the day's jaunt, Elaine came smack upon a challenging hill climb followed by a somewhat risky descent.

Gingerly, she negotiated them in the trusty Mallard. Her reward was an ideal campsite, bordering the creek in an area cooled by the wind.

I didn't know this at the time. Following her up and down the hill, I wondered what she was going to say when I caught up with her. She'd probably tell me what an idiot I was to suggest this risky frontage road.

As I approached the spot where Elaine had/was parked by the creek side, she said, "If you stop here for the day, I have a special treat for you."

Elated at not getting chewed out, I replied, "You've got a deal." She escorted me to the motor home and handed me a chocolate milkshake and said, "This is our best camping spot yet."

About 90 minutes after we settled in, George ran by on the adjacent freeway and yelled, "We'll see you tomorrow at the rest stop up the road." He had stuck to I-70 all day.

Early in the evening, Elaine and I had visitors. First came a dozen Boy Scouts and their scoutmaster, all taking a 15-mile bike ride on the frontage road. Minutes later, a farmer in a pickup and towing a trailer stopped to chat, and in the process pointed out Indian ruins on the mountains across from our creek.

Tonight, beneath the mountains, beside the fast-flowing creek, we almost feel like pioneers camping out.

**DAY 34.** Elaine and I regretfully left our idyllic campsite by the creek at 5:30 this morning and headed up the gravel frontage road paralleling I-70/50. Darkness prevented us from taking a last look at the ruins of the Indian moki huts in the sandstone cliffs.

After traveling two miles on the frontage road, we came upon George and Georgia. They had camped just off the freeway. George and I joined up for the day. The Billingsleys were geared to staying on the freeway, and I decided not to expose Elaine to another risky frontage road hill.

I wasn't a happy camper out there on I-70. The thought of spending 25 miles on this race track depressed me, and I kept casting envious glances at the frontage road.

George reported that he has lost 10 pounds so far, as contrasted with my one pound. Recovered from his injuries (shinsplints and knee problems), he is in good spirits but proceeding cautiously.

This morning's work was a long ascent, probably eight or nine miles, through a gorge to the summit of a mountain. When we reached the top, our altimeter showed it as 8100 feet.

Just as we started down the mountain, we met a bicyclist who said he was traveling from Maine to Las Vegas. He had a mountain bike and it was loaded with gear, including an oversize sleeping bag.

He was a young fellow, mid-20s I'd guess, and gave the impression of being on a shoestring budget. He said, "I've stopped to work at several places along the way."

After he departed, I remarked to George, "Something is missing today. No motorist has offered us a ride or help. We've also seen no wildlife. Maybe that's symptomatic of the 65-plus speed frenzy of this highway."

Following the Interstate, we experienced a logistical problem: The exits were few. This meant that we could conceivably have finished our daily stint, then driven 10 miles or more to find an exit. The return to the start tomorrow could also have been complicated.

Luckily, we ended our 26 miles smack at the junction of

Highway 10. A quarter-mile from the exit, we found a flat spot to camp, and an easy starting spot for tomorrow.

We still have not seen a Utah Highway Patrol officer. (Hey, I'm still alert after 26 miles. I was about to write "patrolman" when women's lib whispered in my ear to make it "officer.")

I apparently forgot to bring along the letter informing me that pedestrians are permitted on I-70. I'm still a bit apprehensive that some officer may give us a bad time.

**DAY 35.** Highway 50 is advertised as the "Loneliest Road in America." That's true from Carson City to Salina, Utah. But at that point when the highway combines with I-70, the road gets busy. I wasn't enthralled this cold, windy morning to face a heavy traffic flow.

But unexpectedly, the divided highway ended after two miles. There we entered old Highway 50, a two-lane road.

Then I saw a parallel two-lane road under construction. It was inviting blacktop. I ventured over to run on it and soon encountered the project foreman. He told me, "It's okay to run here except for the two-mile area where we're working. The new road goes on for 32 miles."

I had this road all to myself, the first person to ever run on it! George, by nature of his being a late riser, got second place.

Running with no cars to worry about and on a smooth surface, I was transcended to hog heaven. King of the road!

As I ran the new road, dozens of cars jockeyed for space on nearby Highway 50. A Utah Highway Patrol officer—the first I'd seen—passed by and paid no attention to me. A good sign.

Later, an officer was across the road from me giving a ticket. He, too, took no notice of me. The fates are kind!

Counted four Greyhound buses today. Guess the strike must be over. Hard to keep in contact with the news out here in the desert.

Atop San Rafael Knob today, after a two-hour uphill pull, I turned around for the view and heard myself saying, "God, You made it so beautiful!"

I was referring to the valley of brilliant red with some blue-grey tints, to the sandstone cliffs of varying hues and designs, and to the snowcapped mountains as a backdrop to all this. Breathtaking scenery. The Utah Tourist Bureau calls this part of Utah "Panoramaland," and justifiably so.

We lucked out in that our 25-mile mark coincided with a rest stop at San Rafael Knob. We're spending the night at this scenic site.

Some Navajo women, from Arizona they told us, were selling

jewelry here when we arrived. I had no choice, considering the quality and fervor of Elaine's pit-crewing, but to buy her a necklace that caught her eye.

**DAY 36.** Last night's rest area proved to be less than restful for two reasons: a stream of traffic flowed in and out, and the noise from parked trucks with generators constantly running.

I returned this morning to the new, unopened I-70 and had it all to myself. As I ran along, taking in all the majestic scenery, my thought was that this area is a textbook of geology. Regrettably, I'm not educated in the language in which it is written.

Another thought: What we need, for the health of the country, is a three- to four-foot blacktop trail taking in many of the nation's scenic wonders—a trail that extends from the Pacific to the Atlantic. Ninety percent of it could be along existing highways. It could be labeled as the "National Fitness Trail," with every mile marked.

Many people would consider the idea of a National Fitness Trail extravagant. But its cost would be minuscule compared to the cost of space, social-service, or drug-abuse programs.

Few aspects of national life are more precious than the health of our people. Such a trail would promote fitness by inspiring people to hike or bike across a state, for example.

I've made a practice of noting thoughts such as these on a miniature tape recorder that I carry while running. This recorder has recently experienced a resurrection.

A couple of days ago before heading out at 5:30 a.m., I attended to a bladder matter in the motor home. Just as I finished in the darkness, Elaine said, "What's was that big plop sound?" I replied, "That was the top of the toilet seat crashing down."

I wasn't on the road five minutes before realizing that the recorder was missing. I figured I'd left it on the dining seat of the motor home.

At the first pit stop, I asked Elaine about it. "Remember that big plop this morning?" she said. "That was your tape recorder crashing into the toilet."

Then she told of bravely extracting it, piece by piece, and letting the car heater blow air on the parts and batteries to dry them. After they dried, she reassembled the recorder.

We played with it for a day, trying to get it to work, but it was unresponsive. But on the second day it showed signs of life again. It now functions with 75-percent efficiency.

This morning, we wended our way through sandstone passes. I felt almost guilty to be all alone on the unopened road while all the traffic competed for space on old Highway 50.

Alas, at four miles I came to an insurmountable obstacle. The new highway dead-ended at a canyon with a 200-foot drop where a bridge was in the initial stages of construction. My only course of action was to detour onto the old highway and cross its bridge.

That done, I returned to the unopened highway. My good fortune ended at seven miles, when the road again became a freeway awash with traffic on both sides.

A Utah Highway Patrol Mustang executed a U-turn on the center divider near me. I was relieved that the officer paid no attention to me.

Elaine later reported, "That officer stopped to talk to me when I was parked and asked if I needed help." She told him our RUNXUSA story.

He left saying, "More power to you and good luck!" And so disappeared most of our apprehension about running on I-70. Nonetheless, I should have brought the clearance letters. There's always one guy who doesn't get the word.

I assessed my injury status today. Seems I have four potentials: (1) the bone on the outside metatarsal of my left foot; (2) left hip joint; (3) left knee which stopped me from running most of January; (4) right groin.

I suspect that (1) and (2) could possibly be arthritic. From time to time, each of these injuries is irritating—none debilitating, but always a cause for concern.

At 23 miles, we looked down from atop a mountain. The view was dramatic: red lava castles, sandstone formations, cliffs, canyons, gorges, and far away a range of mountains with snow.

But a strong wind was stirring up here, and Elaine was anxious to get the motor home away from what could have been dangerous conditions. I told her, "Go until you feel safe, regardless of how far."

Going down the seven-mile descent, I worried about her and the Mallard. The last gorge was sheer rock, 300 feet or so high on both sides, with the wind gusting through it.

Elaine didn't stop until 30-plus miles, making this one of our longest days. By the time I reached her, my quads felt as if I'd run a couple of the canyons in the Western States 100-mile trail race.

Jokingly I told Elaine, "Now that we've done 30 miles, how

about some more days like this?" She threatened to send me to bed without dinner.

Could be worse. She could threaten to send me to bed without her!

**DAY 37.** Georgia Billingsley drove past me shortly before six o'clock this morning. This meant that George had started earlier than usual and was probably not far behind me.

He caught up with me around 15 miles and was bubbling over about the spectacular scenery of yesterday. "I've promised myself that when I get home I'm going to study the geology of this area," he said.

I asked if he wanted to settle for 20 miles today, considering yesterday's 30-miler and the renewed flare-ups of his shinsplints and knee problems. "No way," he said. "Let's try to keep ahead of schedule."

The plan was to restock our provisions in Green River. However, this being a Sunday in Utah and also Memorial Day weekend, we were worried that the grocery stores would be closed.

Elaine made an advance reconnaissance into Green River and returned with a report. I was impressed with what she'd accomplished: she'd checked us in at an RV park, done the laundry, visited the post office, bought the groceries (limited to the meager offerings of the one convenience store that was open), and even made copies of our 1000-mile status report that we are mailing to some friends who asked to be kept informed as we go along. She also reported that the town is abundantly stocked with motels and restaurants.

I wondered if one of them was a pizza parlor. I was whipping up a craving for pizza.

This piling up running mileage is like pregnancy. You crave certain foods.

Atop a hill this morning, I looked back toward the plateau from whence we had come, and the morning sun shone glowingly on the red sandstone. Pausing on the hill, I realized how much safer it was to be on the new I-70 facing traffic than to be on the old Highway 50.

On I-70, I saw the approaching cars, and the breakdown lane was all mine, and a car's width. It suddenly occurred to me that there were three lanes on this north side of the divided highway. Two belonged to cars, one belonged to me. To quote an old Ethel Merman song, "Who could ask for anything more?"

I'd estimate that 75 percent of the approaching truck drivers move over to the left lane when they see me. I wave a friendly greeting to each of them.

One type never gives an inch—the drivers of cattle trucks. Sure wish they would—not so much for the space and safety, but to put some distance between me and the overwhelming odor, plus an occasional drizzle of cattle urine.

Despite this, I'm getting to be a real softie. Every time I see a truckload of cattle being hauled to market, I feel sorry for them. They've had such a short life, they ask so little, and they offend no one.

Unrelated thought: Years ago, I read a story about a horse thief in Oklahoma who was about to be hanged. The hangman told him, "The execution will take place as soon as you speak your last words and no sooner." Whereupon the thief continued to speak for two-and-a-half days.

That's the kind of a running pace I am trying to develop—an outlaw pace, meaning that as long as I continue to run, at any pace, I won't be executed. And if I make it to the state border, I'm a free man. Ah yes, I do fantasize out here in the desert!

Today, a horde of gnats used me as their target range. Damn nuisance.

At the pit stop, I doused myself with insect repellent to combat the gnats. Sprayed with Off, Aspercreme, and Coppertone, I'm a mobile drug store.

Before beginning the run, I had expected that I'd be heavy on Tylenol, Advil, Motrin, or Bufferin to offset stiffness. Not so. Since starting, I've taken a total of four Bufferins and one allergy pill.

Crossing the Green River which gives the town its name, George and I were impressed by the river's size and flow. It looks out of place in this sand-and-gravel setting. The tourist literature told us that the town is a major put-in point for boat trips.

We ran on east of town before driving back here for the night. I was anxious for the day's running to end—not because I was tired but because I couldn't wait to indulge in the creature comforts of the RV park.

We treated ourselves to dinner in a restaurant—opting for Mexican food instead of the pizza I'd craved earlier in the day. Rather than unhook the motor home's electricity, water, sewer, we walked to dinner. Just what I need after a 25-mile day!

**DAY 38.** The terrain east of Green River isn't eye-catching. In fact, it's downright dismal—sand, parched clay, some tumbleweeds, and hills of gravel-sand combination.

Because the sights remain singularly unexciting—with none of the dazzling desert colors or spectacular designs of yesterday—we might have called it a day of nothingness, just covering the distance. Except for George's find.

Let me say before recounting this major event that we often spot objects on the road. Today, I saw a new bar of Sweetheart soap, a pair of jockey shorts, a comb, and 10 sticks of wax.

Coins often catch our eye. This morning, I found a buffalo-head nickel on the road.

A short time later, George gave me the electrifying news that he'd found $135 in a money clip alongside the road. I was happy for him, but more happy over the deal we had made prior to starting the run.

We'd agreed to split all money found. Easiest $67.50 I ever made!

Later, I found a dime. George snickered when I offered him his 50 percent.

The reason he saw the money and I didn't was that he had chosen to run with traffic on the divided highway, while I faced traffic on the other side. When he joined me on my side, we found no more money. Greatest argument I've heard yet for running with traffic!

The Memorial Day traffic was unpleasantly heavy, maybe because we were close to the recreational area of Green River. The headwind blew at least 30 miles per hour and when vehicles, especially trucks, approached at 65 or more, the wind they whipped up slapped us—even driving us back a step or two at times.

After observing dozens of mammoth motor homes (like the $40,000-plus jobs), I came to a conclusion today: 75 percent of them tow a car. In many cases, we are talking about $80,000 or more on wheels rolling down the highway.

A Utah Highway Patrol officer stopped to check us out. After making the usual inquiries, he told us, "Enjoy yourselves," and drove off in his slick white Mustang. Within five minutes, a sheriff's deputy came by and we went through the same routine all over again.

Our camping spot tonight is exactly where we finished the day's run. We simply pulled into the highway median and set up housekeeping. There was nowhere else to go. We're about 40 yards from either road, just parked out on flat, parched clay.

The trick now is to ignore the surroundings and try to get a good night's sleep to face tomorrow. As mentioned a few days ago, I'm now to the point where getting up in the morning and cranking out 25 to 26 miles is much like going to work.

Every day continues to be hard work; there are no easy days. But while I'm sometimes weary, I'm not hurting. For that, I continue to be amazed and thankful.

**DAY 39.** We were awakened at midnight by rain. It signaled that we had to move the motor home, because if the sandy/clay surface we were parked on got water-soaked, we would be stuck.

So we drove to the breakdown lane of I-70 and spent the rest of the night there. The rain, the howling wind and the cars passing nearby—plus being parked at an angle because of the road's tilt—made for a restless night.

We launched at five o'clock this morning in heavy rain, the first since leaving California. I felt encumbered by my rainproof clothing.

The morning's radio reports predicted rain for the next three days in this area. No choice but to keep going.

I shed the rain gear at today's last pit stop—and promptly got soaked in a hailstorm. The motor home now looks like a laundry as Elaine attempts to dry my gear.

While running through the hailstorm, I had to remind myself, "I am enjoying this!"

I was grateful that the rain ceased during our last six miles. We finished under a bright blue sky in which puffy white cumulus clouds floated like dirigibles.

A highway maintenance worker stopped to ask the standard questions and got the standard answers about RUNXUSA. He suggested, "Down I-70 a few miles, leave I-70 and get on the old Highway 50 to Fruita and Grand Junction. I promise you that it's more scenic and the traffic is nil."

At the next pit stop, I reported this news to Elaine. She was anxious to try the alternate route.

A gentleman driving a Titan motor home—that's a biggie—pulled up to ask if I needed help. Give him the Good Guy Award, for he's the first motor home driver to make such an offer in almost 1000 miles.

Odd thought for today: I wonder why there are so many audio cassettes alongside the highway. I see a dozen or more each day. Similarly, a lot of keys seem to get dropped on the road.

Today's terrain was rolling sandhills and flatlands, both with sagebrush barely a foot high. Hardly exciting. Tomorrow should be better with some travel on old Highway 50 and an overnight stay in Fruita on the other side of the Colorado line.

# E S S A Y

## *The Innovator*
### by Dr. Albert J. Sessarego

*(Dr. Sessarego, now retired as superintendent of the Sacramento City Unified School District, keeps busy these days working as a consultant in education and devoting time and energy to Rotarian projects. He stays in good shape by walking, playing tennis, swimming and golfing. He also has taken more than 50 cruises. — Paul Reese.)*

The blizzard that suddenly struck the Sierra Nevadas was the worst September storm in recent memory, and the phones in my office were ringing incessantly. I called for Paul Reese to come downstairs to assist me in allaying the concerns of parents whose children were several miles into the mountains on the school district's first innovative program of my new administration.

"Tell them not to be unduly concerned," stated Paul. "Their leader knows that high country like he knows the back of his hand. Those kids will not only be safe, but they will have an enjoyable experience and learn something. In any case, I will take some people up to the jumping-off place, and go in and see if any help is needed."

It wasn't. The children came tramping out of the hills in excellent shape—relating how they had built lean-to's and snow shelters, learned how to conserve body heat, how to use trees, mountains, and streams as navigational guides, and even how to prepare hot meals in snow country.

Paul subscribed to the military axiom that, in any given regiment, it is probable that "somebody can play the accordion." Accordingly, he found that he need not go abroad to find the experts he needed to lead the more than two-score outdoor and indoor innovative programs—from backpacking to water ballet—that he administered. Expertise in almost every field existed within the personnel ranks of this school district—one of the largest in California.

Paul first came to the Sacramento City Unified School District in 1940 as a teacher. He left the next year to join the Marine Corps.

After retiring from the Corps in 1963, he returned to the school district and served with me in an administrative capacity when I was assistant superintendent. He later was placed in charge of the seven junior highs and five middle schools, a position he held until his retirement in 1981.

As I was preparing to assume the duties of superintendent of schools, Paul and I found ourselves in agreement on two important issues: First, there was a need for education in the wise use of leisure time. Second, the location of our school district at the confluence of two major rivers, adjacent to two large lakes and a deep-water channel, 80 miles from the Pacific Ocean and 50 miles from the Sierra Nevada range, offered unsurpassed opportunities to put theory into practice.

Paul's imagination was unrestricted, and the result was a curriculum of innovative programs that drew inquiries from far and wide. Each program was meticulously structured. There were no simple field trips. They became adventures. It didn't surprise me, then, when Paul himself embarked on the ultimate adventure trip.

# Overview of Colorado

**May 30 to June 17, 1990 — 468.1 miles — 1471.1 total**

| Day | Overnight | Miles | Notes |
|-----|-----------|-------|-------|
| 40 | Fruita | 25.5 | last 14.4 miles in Colorado, completed 1000 miles |
| 41 | nr. Grand Jct. | 25.2 | |
| 42 | near Delta | 25.0 | winds of 40 MPH-plus |
| 43 | near Montrose | 26.1 | temperature down to 25 degrees |
| 44 | Cimarron | 25.0 | |
| 45 | Lake Mesa | 27.7 | |
| 46 | Parlin | 27.8 | |
| 47 | e. of Sargents | 23.4 | temperature 28 |
| 48 | Salida | 25.0 | crossed Continental Divide, temperature 29 |
| 49 | near Coaldale | 25.3 | |
| 50 | Royal Gorge | 25.0 | |
| 51 | near Penrose | 26.4 | |
| 52 | Pueblo | 25.7 | |
| 53 | Fowler | 26.2 | parted with George |
| 54 | Sugar City | 26.0 | |
| 55 | Haswell | 26.1 | |
| 56 | Eads | 26.3 | |
| 57 | Sheridan Lake | 26.1 | |

(first 15.4 miles in Colorado on Day 58)

## Chapter 4

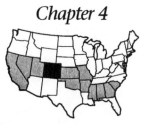

# *Colorado's Ups and Downs*

We'd go over the top in Colorado. Monarch Pass would literally be the high point of the trip at 11,312 feet. Approaching it, we worried as much about the health of our motor homes as our own physical soundness.

Entering our fourth state, I began getting clues from George Billingsley that we would go our separate ways. He preferred a more direct route than the one I'd charted.

We'd be closing in on the halfway point after putting the 468 miles of Colorado behind us between May 30 and June 17. Lots of ups and downs lay between us and that milestone.

**DAY 40.** How do I feel after 1000 miles? Like I've chopped a lot of wood. With 2000 more to go, I realize how much wood is left to chop.

Last night when I stretched in bed, my right knee made a snapping sound and began to hurt. The sharp pain continued for a half-hour or so, then throbbed off and on for the rest of the night. Consequently, I started worried this morning. But as I eased into the run, to my great relief all went well.

Still, my legs felt tired all day. I never can figure this energy-cycle business.

We took the highway maintenance worker's advice and followed old Highway 50 into Fruita, Colorado. George and Georgia elected to stay on the Interstate, saying it was shorter and less hilly and they were not sure of the old road's condition.

Once on it, I immediately encountered ominous signs. One read, "Hazardous Road." Another, "No State Maintenance." Billboards dated back 50 years.

Onward to adventure! As Elaine moved ahead of me, I

wondered how she would react to these conditions. At the next pit stop, she exclaimed her delight with this road and the almost nonexistent traffic.

We stopped to do some camcording at the old border monument which still stands—remarkably without graffiti. A few yards down the road, I passed a dead deer beside the road. Think of the odds against that deer getting hit by a car on a road which probably sees a total of 10 cars on a busy day.

I passed by what had once been a service station, now burned completely. Behind it were two outhouses, both still intact (hey, now we know a safe place in a fire!), and nearby the remains of what had once been a cafe.

I-70 brought the demise of this onetime oasis. A bit of history lies strewn on the ground.

What a shame this road is not maintained better. It could be an excellent bicycle area out of Fruita and Grand Junction— or just a scenic driving route.

We met a total of three cars the entire time on this old highway. In one of them were two senior couples who were lost, having taken a wrong turn out of Fruita. We directed them back to I-70.

It has been a thoroughly delightful day for us. We saw abundant wildlife and were able to scan the scenery without having to be on the lookout for approaching cars. Elaine could drive slowly smack down the middle of the road, and I could run alongside the motor home and visit with her.

There was nothing here but the road, the sound of the wind, the motor home, the birds chirping, the desert, and us. With these kinds of road conditions the whole way, a run across the USA would be a Sunday picnic.

All the way to Mack, a hamlet on the west edge of Colorado, old Highway 50 passed through sandy, sagebrush knolls. Mack is another hamlet killed by I-70, and the remains of a motel, a cafe, and an RV park are evident.

Seventy-five percent of the housing is now mobile homes, and most of them have a dog guarding them. The meanest dog in town, a chained pit bull, lunged in my direction. I prayed his chain would hold. Nearby was a Doberman, not restrained and watching me closely—but not as closely as I watched him.

At the I-70 junction in Mack, we were surprised to run into George and Georgia. George reported, "When I entered Colorado on the Interstate, a sign read 'No pedestrians,' so we got off here at the next exit."

We finished the day together and headed into Fruita for provisions and an RV park. Fruita is misspelled Spanish (it should be "fruta") for "fruit," which this valley, with its many fresh-water streams, has been producing for more than 100 years. The town is located near the Colorado National Monument, a scenic wonder and popular tourist attraction.

**DAY 41.** Sunrise this morning was sensational. The sun peeked up over the mountain range and focused on the red cliffs to the south, highlighting their many colors.

After seeing no trees for many miles, I was impressed with the number of trees in Fruita. A tree that I would not give a second glance in California suddenly seems gigantic here. Fruita is touted as a fruit-raising area, but I passed through the entire area without seeing a single orchard.

George came by early this morning, driving to his start. He stopped to say, "Georgia and I are going to stay on the trail all day." This meant they wouldn't interrupt the run to tour the Colorado National Monument.

Elaine and I took time out to visit the monument, which preserves one of the great landscapes of the American west. The plateau and canyon country, with its towering masses of naturally sculptured rock, embrace 32 square miles of rugged terrain.

We didn't have good luck with the tour. After driving a short part of it, we had to abort the trip. Extensive construction would involve several 30-minute delays, and we didn't have that kind of time. Also, the steep, narrow road was a strain on the motor home, and we were depending on its health to carry us through our trek.

The road I ran today was a big letdown after the solitude of the old abandoned highway. Today's Highway 6, a two-laner between Fruita and Grand Junction, is a veritable racetrack.

The motorists drove with a vengeance, and none offered a ride or help. It's obvious we're in Colorado now. In Utah, I would have had at least a dozen offers.

I gave these drivers a wide berth. On this narrow road without a shoulder, I had to jump into the weeds so many times I'm due to be sprayed with Roundup to de-weed.

Oh, the wisdom: Colorado prohibits pedestrians on I-70 and permits them on this two-lane road. Yet the Interstate is much safer than this suicide alley.

Grand Junction brought us back onto divided Highway 50. But it gave no relief from the sound and fury of traffic that had frustrated me all day. I was just scratching out the miles.

**DAY 42.** We launched our day, again at 5:30 a.m., in a cheerless area of rolling hills, sagebrush, sand, and clay soil. Barren.

The wind blew at 25 miles per hour at the start and increased to 40 or more as the day wore on. Naturally it was a headwind, and sometimes just walking against it was difficult.

I would like to have had an anemograph to measure the wind velocity as the big trucks went by me at 65 MPH and the wind blew toward me at a minimum of 40. Each time I had to brace myself, and still they pushed me back a couple of feet.

I continue to be impressed with the courtesy of Utah drivers. All the cars that moved over today to give me some running space had Utah plates, as did the only three trucks to yield. I'd consider it a miracle if anyone from Colorado moved over.

As a woman driver approached, she seemed to be staring. She even drove over the white fog line to get a closer look. Next time, I'll charge admission!

On a serious note, I experienced the scariest incident to date. I was rounding a corner on a ledge with a 150- to 200-foot dropoff. The road had absolutely no shoulder, only a foot or so of road edging. The wind was blowing 40 to 50 miles an hour, pushing me all over the road.

I saw two semi trucks approaching. They couldn't move over because cars were in the fast lane.

I was already having trouble staying on the road because of the wind. The force of these semis passing by would most likely push me over the edge of the road and onto the dropoff.

Sizing up the situation, I realized that an instant decision was in order. I dived for the edge of the road and laid down there next to the ledge in order to be off the road and to nullify the blowing by the trucks.

Seeing all this, the truck drivers gave me what few inches they could. The trucks passed perilously close, and I heard the deafening thrump of the tires and felt their warmth.

Shaking from the experience, I scrambled up and ran 50 yards down the road to the safety of a guardrail. I hugged the rail as if it were my security blanket and tried to rid myself of the heebie-jeebies.

Relatively composed again, I headed down the road, thanking God I was still numbered among the living. Then a thought crossed my mind: If I had been killed, I hope people would have realized that I died doing what I wanted to do, that I went out enjoying. To me, that would be a helluva lot more delightful death than lingering months in some bed, home, or hospital, then dying, evaporated in body and mind from my usual self.

All in all, this has been one of those days when it has been hard for me to remember, "I'm enjoying." Tonight as I write the final lines on this day, I'm reflecting on our trek that is now one-third of its way along.

Conceptually, in the aggregate, it seems overwhelming—almost insurmountable. But attacked on a day-to-day basis, it is conquerable. The trick is to take it one day at a time. The good days are certain to offset the bad.

**DAY 43.** Each day on the road is a random collection of sights, sounds, experiences, thoughts, and feelings which I sort out each night. Today, in the interest of realism and variety, I report these impressions as they come to me and in the present tense.

As we drive west of Delta to start this early morning hour, I can clearly see the silhouettes of all the mountain ranges that surround this valley. The ranges to the southeast have snow on them.

This is a different world from yesterday. There is no rampaging wind, no rain, and little traffic. Kind of wish I'd gotten out here an hour earlier.

My left foot sends a signal that it is a bit out of sorts from having been at a 30-degree angle most of yesterday. I'm forcing the pace a bit, trying to make time under these good conditions.

In the darkness I hear a noise ahead, then recognize it as a car approaching. Another brilliant Colorado driver with no headlights.

Now a second Colorado driver goes by without headlights. Guess this is some sort of a macho thing.

I'm on a newly paved section of Highway 50, but there's one omission: no shoulder. Questionable economy, even for car and driver safety. What choice does a driver with a car breakdown have but to park on the road?

Colorado drivers approaching me this morning have the entire road to themselves, yet they refuse to move over even one foot for me. I can't figure out whether this results from a lack of courtesy or a lack of intelligence. I can figure, though, that they'd all benefit from a driver training course in Utah or Nevada.

What's this, a car actually moving over for me? Oh, it carries New Mexico plates.

Now here's something just short of a miracle. A guy driving a station wagon with a Colorado license just moved over, and he even waved. Must be a runner. I hereby nominate him for governor!

Hallelujah! I just picked up a three-foot-wide bike path.

Into Delta. I have nothing but kind words for the town which sort of reminds me of how towns were 20 or 30 years ago. Extremely neat and clean, and tree-lined.

It's evident from all the motels and restaurants that there is reliance here on tourist trade. Yet it's a town designed to accommodate the local population.

As I go by McDonald's, I suddenly acquire a taste for hot cakes. Detour across the street to pick up an order and eat it as I move along. A bit gooey with the syrup dripping.

Delta advertises itself as the "City of Murals." My favorite mural is Ute County, which depicts Indians, buffalo and an Indian encampment. Elaine and I take time out to camcord it.

East of Delta, Highway 50 becomes a divided road with a wide shoulder and this happy happenstance continues all the way to Montrose. Manna from heaven!

Today is surprising in that I anticipated desert terrain and a two-lane road without a shoulder. Instead, we find a green belt and a four-lane highway.

Up ahead, the road curves to the right and appears headed for the snow-laden mountains. Tilt! Are those on our route?

Elaine and I detour from Highway 50 to tour Olathe, a town once on the main road and now suffering from being bypassed. The business buildings now stand empty. On the outskirts of Olathe is a worm farm which I don't have time to tour.

Last stop, Montrose. It is home of the Black Canyon, one of Colorado's scenic wonders.

After studying the road configuration, we decide the canyon route is too hilly and curvy for the motor home. We stick with Highway 50.

I finish running, and we treat ourselves to a frosty at Wendy's. Between that and pampering ourselves with RV creature comforts, a wild time is had by all!

**DAY 44.** At 32 degrees with a wind-chill factor, it was a bit cold starting out this morning. I had to run with some vigor to keep from freezing.

The day later warmed up to 60 or 70 degrees, requiring several wardrobe changes. The process is becoming standardized.

I start with a polypropylene top and lycra tights under a lined windbreaker suit, plus gloves and a knit cap. At my first pit stop, I trade the lined suit for an unlined one, and the knit cap for a ball cap. The gloves come off, but I continue to carry them dangling from my fanny pack.

Then at the second pit stop, I usually change to a T-shirt and half-tights or shorts. The fanny pack always stays, as does the headgear for sun protection. Since the weather is so suddenly changeable, I usually carry a windbreaker draped from the fanny pack.

My bandanna has become another invaluable accessory. It keeps the sun off the back of my neck and protects my cut lips. Besides, it gives me a rather rakish appearance.

George Billingsley reappeared today. We ran the last 20 miles together.

We encountered a young bicyclist from Yorkshire, England, who was traveling from the east. He gave us a good description of what lay ahead: plenty of hillwork. Leaving Montrose, we ran steadily uphill toward Cerro Summit.

Signs along the road advertised Black Canyon Monument. By now, I've learned that "monument" is misleading since it usually connotes an edifice of some type. Colorado monuments such as Black Canyon extend over hundreds of acres of spectacular scenery.

Outside of town, our road narrowed to two lanes but had a good bike lane. As we started up the pass, farms lined both sides of the highway. The setting conveyed an atmosphere of tranquility. But this was soon shattered by seeing several drivers passing dangerously over the double-yellow lines.

This brought up the question, "What can be done to discourage reckless driving?" Then came an inspiration: "Once a Highway Patrolman arrests a reckless driver, the procedure should not be to issue him a ticket and then let him drive off. Instead, the driver's car should be impounded on the spot for at least 24 hours. Now that would create some dramatic scenarios."

At the 7958-foot summit, I was surprised to see a small ranch. Hundreds of sheep grazed nearby. To the north towered a Rocky Mountain range, and to the south, smaller mountains covered with greenery.

The scenery today has been quite a contrast to the previous two or three days. It has been uphill and downhill all day—mountains covered with grass, small sagebrush, and plants resembling manzanita but a little more willowy. With all the mountain passes up and down, it has been one of those days when I'm eager to find out what's around the next corner.

We lucked out with our finish, stopping only a mile from a small RV park located directly on Cimarron Creek and under a grove of trees. George and Georgia anchored nearby.

The fast-flowing creek, the trees, and the mountain backdrop add up to a serene and picturesque setting. In fact, this setting is the major excitement of the day.

**DAY 45.** We started today in the bowels of a valley surrounded by magnificent cliffs. A few nearby hills had snow on them.

This was a cheerful valley with several farms scattered throughout it and plentiful water. Cimarron Creek itself resembled a small river.

Highway 50 hugged the mountain on the north side. On the south was a broad valley so picture-book perfect that I expected to see it laced with a golf course.

George and I ran the first few miles together early this morning. He said his weight loss is now 15 pounds. He added, "I don't think I'm eating enough."

I couldn't argue with that. My weight fluctuation has never been more than three pounds.

Our major obstacle today was Blue Mesa, an 8650-foot summit. As usual when I cross through a pass like this, the wind was strong. It reminded me of running the 36-mile Run to the Sun Race on Maui. Going up to the Haleakala Crater, we were battered by the wind at each turn.

On our way to the summit today, we encountered the roughest highway construction so far on our trip: a half-mile of rock and gravel. The cars and trucks passing raised a dust storm and sent small chunks of gravel flying.

We spotted a UPS truck at the summit. I'm beginning to think that they might deliver to the Matterhorn.

I ran down the summit faster than I've run in a long spell. It will be interesting to see if this affects me tomorrow. But it was a fun thing to do and, Lord, I felt good doing it.

While concentrating on the descent, I was startled to hear somebody yell, "How you doing?" I looked to my right to see a bicyclist approaching me from the rear.

"Where are you going?" I hollered. "Chicago," he replied.

"And you?" he asked. "Savannah," I told him.

We talked a short while, wished each other good luck, and moved off at our different speeds. Seeing how fast he went, I thought again that maybe I should be biking instead of running. With that thought came the corollary: If I were biking, oh, my aching arse!

Later, I met a young bicyclist from Minneapolis on his way to the California redwoods. Seeing him got me to thinking about the merits of a college summer course designed around biking across the USA, or parts of it, and studying sociology, geography, geology, and such.

This would make a helluva lot more sense than many college courses these days. The trip would be a lifetime experience, and the log kept would be a lifetime memory.

Elaine reported having a conversation with a woman in Sapinero who'd asked her "to talk a bit." The woman told Elaine that recently three different types of USA trekkers had passed by here: a unicyclist, a roller skater and a paraplegic. I couldn't feature any of them making it up some of the hills, but I guess they found a way.

'Tis another day in Colorado with no offers of a ride or help. But do note that I have refrained from commenting on Colorado's drivers. Yes, this does take restraint.

Elaine and I lived it up tonight by dining at Pappy's Restaurant at the lake marina. Blue Mesa Lake is the largest body of water in Colorado, stretching 20 miles and covering over 10,000 acres when full. It is in this setting that we are camped tonight.

**DAY 46.** Today, my thoughts turned to motor homes. For want of entertainment, I counted 82 of them at the Blue Mesa RV Park. Sixty-two more at the Sunnyside RV Park a short distance later.

Stevens Creek RV Park, a national park site, housed only 20 motor homes. The reason was simple: no hookups. The National Park Service obviously needs to modernize.

As I continue to observe this endless parade of motor homes, I conclude that Detroit automobile magnates are missing a great bet. Have they studied the motor home market? Instead of just making the truck engine and frame, as with our Chevy 350 for the Mallard, Detroit could produce the whole ball of wax—engine, frame, motor home—and realize big profits.

Big news of the day: A farmer pulled out of his driveway and offered a ride. Hey, that was a first for Colorado!

Today's route took us to and through Gunnison. Once again, we were blessed with good weather. The sky, a powder blue, was absolutely clear. Even the wind was kind until afternoon.

The scenic pattern for the entire day consisted of a pass through foothills, a green and fertile valley given over to farming, a pass, a valley. Every three miles or so in this recreational area, there was a picnic or camping site.

Let's describe today's scenery this way: all very pleasant and interesting, but none of it merited camcording.

As I approached Gunnison from the west, small farms gave way to the usual series of motels, auto dealers, motorcycle dealers and storage facilities. Gunnison itself surprised me. I'd expected to find it among hills, but it's in a flat area.

I walked through the downtown area, while Elaine took time out to buy groceries, do laundry, and visit the post office. I checked bookstores and a visitors' center for Monarch Pass maps, and came away with some useful information on the pass that looms two days ahead.

I learned that Monarch is eight miles up from Sargents, tomorrow's destination. The road over the pass has no bike lane but does offer a wide dirt shoulder as compensation.

Today was without any major climbs or descents. I tried to take it easy, saving my juice for Monarch.

**DAY 47.** George and I linked up again today, and we both confessed to feeling an undercurrent of excitement as we closed in on Monarch Pass. It was 28 degrees when we started this morning at an elevation of 8400 feet. Just how cold will it be on the pass, which is at 11,312 feet?

The scenery throughout this day was constant: a green, fertile valley enclosed on the south side by small mountains with some tree growth, and on the north side by sand and sagebrush hills. Pass after pass unfolded the same scene.

All the way from Parlin to the beginning of the Monarch Pass grade, intervening hills masked any view of the Monarch range. But the gradual climb to 9100 feet left no doubt what lay ahead tomorrow.

One redeeming feature as we approached Sargents was the relatively light traffic. Sargents is a hamlet with 20 or so structures, one of them named Dotty's Last Stop.

We stopped there to inquire about the distance to the summit (9-1/2 miles) and to any camping spots before the top (only one on the highway, three miles from town). Elaine and Georgia drove ahead to settle in while George and I mushed on.

The camping area consisted simply of parking spaces off a

dirt road that winds through aspens and pines. Elaine and Georgia argued successfully that we make it a short-mileage day and roost here for the night.

Elaine hoped we would be invaded by some wild critters tonight. As she cooked a steak for dinner, I expected a bear or mountain lion to appear for a handout. None came. The only critter on hand this evening is a mosquito that invaded the motor home. Elaine swears it is the size of a grasshopper. I don't see him, but his buzzing reminds me of the Japanese plane in World War II that appeared nightly over Guadalcanal. We called it "Washing Machine Charlie."

**DAY 48.** Today marked the high point to date of our trek. We crossed the Continental Divide via Monarch Pass. Never before had we started so high: 9100 feet. The evergreens were elbow to elbow in this pass, and the cut through the side of the mountain left the road perched on a rocky ledge.

The highway up the pass from the west had no bike lane. But there was a shoulder of gravel approximately three feet wide. But early on, we encountered a problem that recurred at least a half-dozen times. The road made a sharp bend and the shoulder narrowed to 12 inches between the rocky mountain and the very edge of the highway.

I approached these turns unable to see what was coming, and I had to listen intently for vehicles. On two occasions, I was forced to embrace the rocky cliff. At those moments, I was glad I don't have a big rump that would protrude onto the roadway.

Going up this pass reminded me somewhat of running the 28-mile race up and down Pike's Peak. That race starts at about 7,500 feet in Manitou Springs and tops off at 14,108 feet, and then swoops down from the peak back to Manitou.

Strange, I thought today, how that 14,108 figure sticks with me. Guess it's because after you run something like that, you are not likely to forget it.

Thinking of a run like that now, I sort of wonder how I did it. But, again, there's a healthy difference between age 58 (mine at Pike's Peak) and age 73 (my vintage now).

On the way up the Monarch summit, I stopped to play Good Samaritan by removing two rocks—almost soccer-ball size—from the road. All this at the risk of a hernia despite my rolling, not lifting, the rocks.

The climb up to the crest, George and I agreed, was surprisingly easy. Georgia and Elaine were waiting for us at the summit.

Arriving at the crest, George reacted jubilantly. He has, from the beginning of the trip, worried about his motor home making it over Monarch. He bought the motor home with 59,000 miles already on it, so he had qualified confidence in it.

After each day's run, he has checked the oil and water and then kissed it on the hood in appreciation of its performance. Understandably, when it arrived at the summit, he came close to having an affair with it!

Elaine refurbished me with some hot soup. She decided not to ride the Tamrac, which promised views up to 150 miles (including Pike's Peak) and which costs only $4.50. We settled for visiting the gift shop to buy postcards and the *Cookbook for Road Kills.*

George and I were excited about the ease of running down the mountain. Yet we realized we must exercise caution or wind up tired or injured.

A little over a mile down, we passed the Monarch ski area which, from my quick glance, did not appear impressive. A couple of miles down we went by Monarch Lodge, which looked quite comfortable and spacious. Since it provides free shuttle to the ski area, I'd assume it is popular.

A little farther down sat the Monarch cross-country ski area, housed beside an old mine or gravel operation. In either event, not too attractive.

The downhill road from the summit was almost a flip side of the up: about the same gradient, same distance, along the rocky ledge and with tree-studded hills on both sides. Creeks and cascading water appeared often.

On both the up and down roads, there were many turnouts. Elaine and I were appalled at the instances of reckless driving we witnessed—motorists passing over the double-yellow line and cutting in very close. Unfortunately, police seem to consider speeding a more serious offense, which it is not.

At 25 miles, we called it a day because the junction of Highways 50 and 285 made a convenient ending spot. Our campsite is located between a fast-flowing creek and a small lake, under a grove of trees. Very restful.

Why, we can even get the local radio station. The highlight tonight is the reading of students' names from the honor roll.

**DAY 49.** I thought back today on the apprehension we had harbored about Monarch Pass. Yet in the doing it turned out to be relatively easy. There's a lesson to be learned here.

I wasn't feeling any effects of altitude as I jogged along this morning. But my quadriceps were acutely aware of the Monarch trek. They lamented yesterday's rapid descent.

The cushioning of the new shoes I wore today provided some comfort. Maybe I should retire shoes at 400 miles rather than at 525 as planned.

George and I didn't run together all day. I started half an hour before him, and because the Monarch downhill had been unkind to his knee, he didn't catch up with me.

George told me tonight that, battling injury signals, he rotated three pairs of shoes today—Nike Air Mariah, Reebok 2000 PB and Nike Spiridon Gold. Hey, bartender, make mine New Balance 840, dear faithful shoe that it's been!

The day's run descended from 7,036 to 6,200 feet. The approach to Salida passed through a green, fertile valley from which a herd of long-horned cattle stared at me. Down the road a bit, a pasture of bulls showed even more interest. No wonder. I had on a red windbreaker suit.

Mountain ranges around it tower considerably above Salida. As we entered town, I turned around for a last look at the majesty of the Monarch range. The sun shining on the snow intensified its splendor.

Salida boasts that it has the highest concentration of peaks 14,000 feet or more in continental USA. It also enjoys an average of 300 days of sunshine per year.

I went by the city park with a massive building which, I read, held both a hot springs and an indoor swimming pool. Why couldn't I have discovered that last night?

From a distance, I spotted that great symbol of American culture: the Golden Arches. Alas, like most other McDonald's in the small towns, this one wasn't open for breakfast.

I passed the local high school—an adequate-looking plant but not equipped with lights for night football. Probably because it's too cold here at night. Besides, in a town this size, what could be more exciting on a Saturday afternoon than a high-school football game?

East of Salida, Highway 50 began to parallel the Arkansas River, a fast-flowing stream popular with rafters. Besides rafting, horseback riding and mountain biking on trails are big in this part of the country.

Seeing this river made me think: why hasn't someone figured a way to kayak and portage across the USA? Anything is possible. Many years ago, I read in *Life* magazine of a German who had paddled across the Atlantic in a rubber kayak. And if I recall correctly, Lewis and Clark used a rubber boat in at least one of their expeditions.

Back to reality. Elaine reported at a pit stop, "A tornado hit in Limon, Colorado, and blew two semis off the road." Scary, in that our original RUNXUSA course was very close to Limon.

At nine miles, we lost the bike lane that had been with us since the start today. From there on, I hopscotched between the highway and the gravel shoulder, avoiding cars.

Several times today, I encountered a difficult running situation. The highway made "S" turns, and there was only abut 15 inches between the guardrail and the edge of the highway. Often I had to embrace the railing to avoid cars, since the road was banked towards the rail. At those moments, I got vile thoughts about whoever designed this narrow two-lane highway.

We landed for the night near Coaldale, in a pleasant valley with towering peaks to the south and tree-covered mountains to the north and east. Tired as Elaine and I are, the simple amenities of the RV park are comforting.

Monarch yesterday was a milestone. The next will be when we go over 1500 miles in little more than a week from now and consider that as being halfway finished.

**DAY 50.** The start this morning was quite impressive. It took us through a rocky gorge, somewhat narrow, where the cliffs rose 300 feet on either side of the highway. The early morning sun spotlighted through a narrow passage to light the road.

The river was with us all 25 miles today. Its fast-flowing white water makes it a mecca for river rafters.

At several points along the way, Highway 50 drops down as close as four feet from the river. It puzzles me that river overflows don't flood the highway.

For amusement, George and I played fool-around by trying to toss rocks across the Arkansas River. With a grunt-and-groan effort, we succeeded—but barely.

The day turned out to be good and bad. Good in that the river provided much entertainment as rafters negotiated the rapids. Bad because the narrow road, without a shoulder, meant miserable and dangerous running.

Traffic was unusually heavy this morning, probably because it was Saturday and all the people in search of recreation were out and about. All day, cars, pickups and buses towing rubber rafts clogged the highway in both directions.

From beginning to end today, there was no bike lane. Worse yet, much of the road had sharp curves and only a foot or so of space between the highway's edge and the guardrail. Like yesterday, this required stopping often and leaning on the railing to avoid oncoming vehicles.

Ironically, George and I had worried about going up and down Monarch Pass. That was a piece of cake compared to today's tightrope act.

One feature I like about running is that it provides opportunity for meditating. But that I can't do on roads like today's, because if not alert to the traffic I'm liable to get splattered.

After a pit stop where Elaine stuffed me with peach coffee cake, major willpower was needed for me to get started again. Boy, would a short nap have felt nice! Oh hell, as long as I was dreaming, why not make it all day in bed?

Had a scary experience with my right knee—felt as if I were damaging a tendon or ligament. Feeling the pain, I braked to an immediate stop, did some probing and walking, and the knee quickly returned to normal. I was left wondering, "What in hell was that?"

We finished the day in heavy rain and thunder at the south entrance to the Royal Gorge. From our nearby RV park, we can actually see the Royal Gorge Bridge.

At dinner Elaine told me about her extended conversation with an elderly lady who operates a small store near here. The last four years, the woman had said, were the best of her life, because for the previous 20 years she had taken care of her husband, who had Alzheimer's and was extremely mean to her.

"If I had it to do over," she said, "I'd have drowned him in the Arkansas River. Oh well, at least I'm grateful that he's been dead four years."

The woman's custom is to sit outside the store, which is where she was when Elaine met her. If you want something inside, you go in and get it yourself, then come out and pay her. She refuses to move.

She also told Elaine that a couple of days ago she had unknowingly entertained a convict who had escaped from the Canon City prison. The old girl put some spice into Elaine's day.

This is not, it develops, a night to relax. We're told that a tornado watch is in effect for the area, and we damn well know that a motor home is not the place to be in a tornado. Sleep unsoundly!

**DAY 51.** No tornadoes overnight but plenty of rain. The skies this morning threatened more of the same, but none came all day.

George, who'd done extra mileage yesterday so he could sleep in today, met me at two miles. We ran together to the north entrance to Royal Gorge.

Elaine and I then played tourist—while George and Georgia continued the run—and visited the Gorge, which features the world's highest suspension bridge, 1053 feet above the Arkansas River. We were told it attracts a half-million visitors a year.

It's an interesting operation, I learned. The 3500-acre park is a private enterprise. Owned by Canon City, it is in turn leased to a woman from Dallas for $700,000 a year.

Nowhere in all the advertising we saw were the prices listed. We discovered them while driving to the entrance gate. The toll was $4 a person for entrance only. To ride the gondola or train, you paid a heavier fee.

Prohibited from crossing the bridge were campers, motor homes and pedestrians. So much for our preferred modes of travel.

On the road again (Thank ya, Willie!), I immediately saw a world of difference between Highway 50 east of the Royal Gorge and west of it. To the west, Highway 50 had been two narrow, curvy, lanes with no shoulder. To the east, it is three lanes with a bike lane on each side.

The road from Royal Gorge to Canon City was carved between two mountain ranges covered with pine trees, some scrub growth and a reddish soil. Nothing spectacular here.

On the outskirts of Canon City, I passed the Colorado State Penitentiary. It became a state prison in 1876, and some of the structures looked that old.

As I ran through the prison parking lot to stay off the shoulderless highway, I wondered how many guards in the prison towers had their eyes on me. I saw no prisoners in the exercise yard this morning. They were probably all in church, praying for enlightenment on a way to escape.

I was thinking that this was a rough old town when I came across the Chablis Restaurant Francais. Ooh, la, la— sophistication!

In the previous nine days in Colorado, neither Elaine nor I

had had a Colorado Highway Patrolman stop and ask us if we needed help. Contrast that with the Utah Highway Patrol which was very solicitous.

At a pit stop today, the streak was broken. We explained our mission to a courteous and understanding officer. I told him, "You're the first Colorado Highway Patrol officer to inquire." He said that was due somewhat to the patrol being short-handed because of a tight budget.

He explained, "The patrol is not too popular with state legislators. Seems that some have been ticketed. Thinking they had diplomatic status to drive as they want, the legislators resented this and retaliated by whacking our budget."

After listening to him, I hereby retract all previous unkind remarks about the Colorado Highway Patrol.

**DAY 52.** Started this morning, again in darkness, in the Arkansas River Valley. It is an open, grassy area with mountain ranges on each side of the highway, both 15 to 20 miles distant.

Sunrise here is quite different from in the desert of Nevada or in the Utah mountains. It's more diffused. This morning, the sun reflected a scarlet glow on the clouds in the east and painted the clouds to the west a pale pink.

At one point, I went by a sandstone cliff that made it hard to distinguish whether I was in Nevada, Utah or Colorado. The cliff had 25 distinct layers or strata.

My enjoyment of this pastoral setting was dampened considerably by the endless traffic on Highway 50 which is a race track between Canon City and Pueblo. The swirling of traffic is not the kind of music I enjoy.

Let's give this highway due credit, though. It has very little litter. And the same Highway Patrolman who talked with us yesterday stopped again to talk today.

I didn't run with George today since he started three miles ahead of me. He was in a hurry to get into Pueblo to buy some new shoes.

Too much of my day was spent in and around Pueblo, where the population is 104,000 and the navigation was tricky. It involved a mile-and-a-half stretch south on Interstate 25 (which in this area coincides with Highway 50). Since pedestrians are not allowed on Interstates in Colorado, I had to parallel I-25 by following a frontage road, then cut through a grassy area and finally cross a railroad area to reconnect with Highway 50.

This navigation was the only excitement of the day. More exciting for Elaine because she lost me for a while in Pueblo. She had worked on the assumption that I would avoid I-25 entirely and take Highway 47. After traveling that road for five miles and not finding me, she started to hoist the panic flag.

She then stopped to regroup and realized that I had probably followed 50 through town. Driving that way, she quickly found me.

She had some unkind words to say about my moronic routing. Oh well, a day like this makes us appreciate all the good days we've had.

**DAY 53.** On our drive out of Pueblo this morning, Elaine and I agreed that this was one of those towns you couldn't exit too soon.

I was looking forward to departing Highway 50 and getting on a quiet road, Highway 96. After going through Pueblo, I'm glad that our routing avoids big cities as much as possible.

George started two miles ahead of me this morning, so I wasn't sure I would catch him on one of the most important days to date. I found him waiting for me so he could say goodbye. Within an hour, we would take different routes.

Here's the story behind that decision. When I originally laid out our route across the USA, I sought the shortest distance from Jenner, California, to Savannah, Georgia, but with some stipulations: back roads and scenery took precedence over shorter, busier highways.

I briefed George on this philosophy and asked him to review the routing. He said, "That's your department. I agree with whatever you do."

But for the last couple of weeks, George had been considering striking off on a shorter, faster route and suggested that I should follow suit. He expressed reservations about taking Highway 96 out of Pueblo.

He said, "Georgia and I have studied the maps and calculate that, by following Highway 50, we can save 38 miles between the junction of Highways 50 and 96 and Pratt, Kansas."

That was important to him because he and Georgia had now decided they wanted to finish as soon as possible. George felt the need to get home to manage his business affairs. Georgia missed her grandchildren and worried about her elderly father.

George said, "By the combination of taking direct and major highways, and by extending my day a few hours, I can finish several days earlier. Also, Georgia and I both prefer the main highways."

To the contrary, Elaine and I favor the quiet back roads, and we are in no particular hurry to finish. We want to hold to our goal of not less than 25 or more than 27 miles per day. We enjoy our free time together in the afternoon and don't want to lose it by extending our day.

After more than 1,300 miles on the road, George and I each know what we want on and from the run, and our thinking runs in two different directions. I respect his reasons for accelerating, and he respects mine for sticking with the planned route.

On parting, we wished each other the best of luck and set up a system to communicate at Pratt, Kansas, and Hardy, Arkansas. While Elaine will miss Georgia's company, she, too, prefers to follow through as originally planned. Thus it was that, at 8:38 a.m. today, at the junction of Highways 50 and 96, we went our separate ways.

It was a delight to be on a country road again instead of a busy highway. The traffic on 96 was light, and 90 percent of the drivers moved over as they saw me. Unbelievable in Colorado!

I did hook up with new companions today: some sort of horseflies with a nasty bite. The scenario read like this: I'm running, feel a sting, stop, see a horsefly, swat it, my hand is full of blood, and a dead fly drops to the road.

Give the flies credit for one thing. They force me to run. Once I slow to a walk, they use me for a landing pad.

Turns out that our goodbyes to George and Georgia this morning were premature. About two hours after we had settled in at an RV park, the Billingsleys appeared for a farewell rendezvous.

**DAY 54.** When George was running with me, he usually got started at six a.m. This morning, he was on his way at 5:10. I suspect he is hell-bent for mileage.

I cautioned him when we parted yesterday, "You are your own worst enemy. If you get into injury trouble, that will be the cause: overdoing."

The thought crossed my mind early this morning that, in our pre-planning, Elaine and I had thought we'd spend every fifth to seventh night in a motel. But we soon realized that would be foolish for several reasons.

First, it would cost three or four times as much as an RV park. Second, the only attraction at a motel would be a shower, and that we can get at an RV park. Third, a motel involves moving clothes and toiletries from the motor home to the motel room and back, which is a nuisance. Fourth, a motel means sleeping in somebody else's bed instead of our own double bed.

There's also the consideration that, while sleeping in a motel, we leave the motor home unguarded. We need practically everything in it to complete this safari.

The entire day today I ran through the Arkansas River Valley, with not a mountain to be seen in any direction. This contrasted sharply with what we've been used to the last month.

I noted a sign telling me that Limon, scene of the recent tornadoes, was only 76 miles away. Later, I saw a gate made to go across Highway 96. I asked a workman about the gate. He said, "It's to keep cars from traveling on this road when a blizzard is raging."

Tornadoes to the north, blizzards to the east. Great country!

I'm paying a price in extra mileage on this country road (versus George's direct route), but it's well worth it. Most of the time, the road is all mine.

The few drivers here continue to move over voluntarily, and many of them wave to me. Why are farm folks so much more friendly than city dwellers?

I met my first bicyclist in quite a while. He started in Virginia and is headed for Jackson Hole, Wyoming.

He said, "I'm taking it rather leisurely, 50 miles or so a day. I'm not even sure of my route." Once again, I admire these bicyclists who are loaded with gear and self-sufficient.

What I had dreaded the most today didn't materialize: the bombardment by the horseflies. (The first question George asked when he finished his run yesterday was, "Did those horseflies attack you?") I didn't use suntan oil today, so I'm wondering if that attracted them before.

Other problems took the diverse form of dogs, hay, and water. Farm dogs are a persistent problem. There's always the potential that a hungry one will come charging out and want a piece of meat—my flesh!

When farmers drove by with a loose load of hay, the dust transported me to allergy land. And for the first time in 1,350 miles, I had pulled the stupid stunt of forgetting to fill my water bottle at the pit stop.

**DAY 55.** Here was the scene this morning: the highway stretched out all the way to the horizon, open fields on both sides of the road, no mountains visible in any direction.

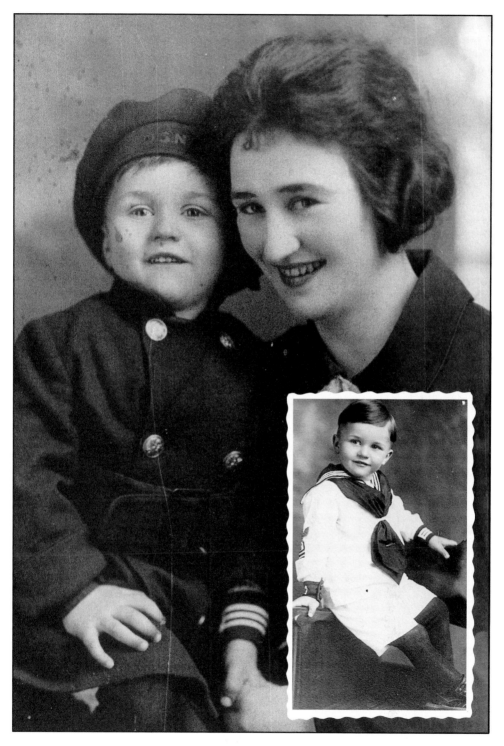

A young Paul Reese with his mother, Elsie Reese; (inset) Paul Reese at age three and a half, 1920–21.
*Credit: Paul Reese Collection*

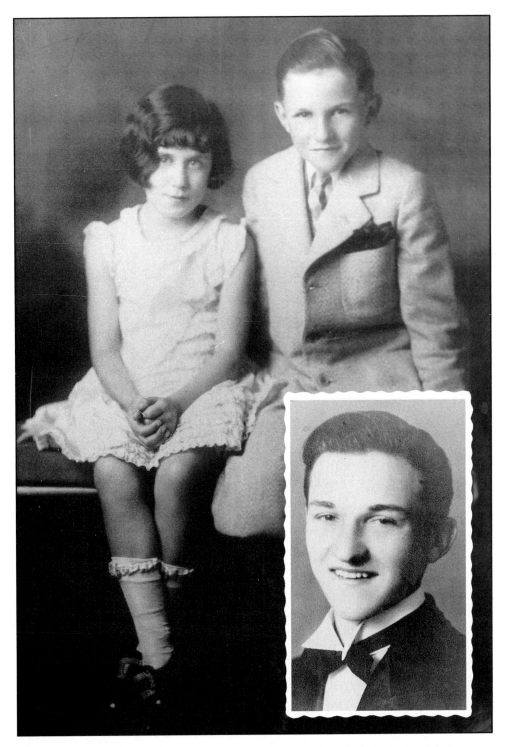

Paul Reese and sister June Reese, grammar school days; (inset) Paul's high school graduation portrait, 1935.
*Credit: Paul Reese Collection*

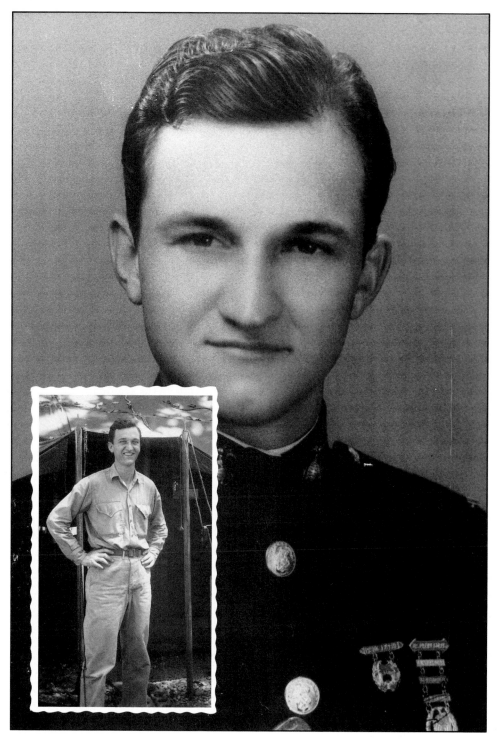

First Lieutenant Paul Reese, USMC, and (inset) Paul at Guadalcanal during WWII.
*Credit: Paul Reese Collection*

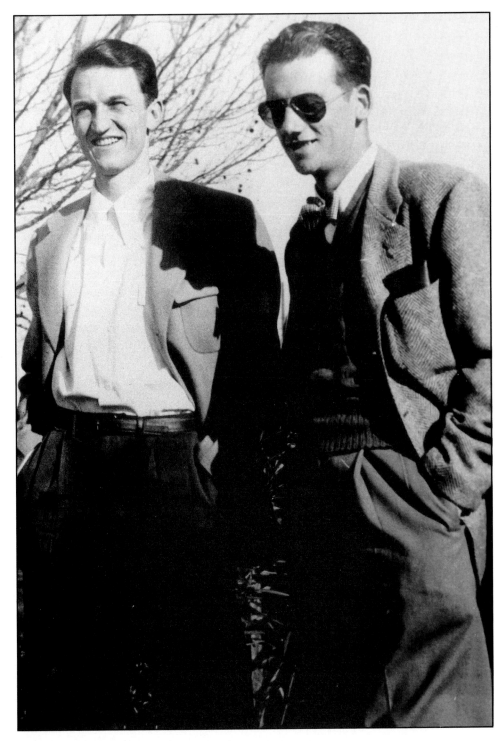

Paul (left) and Bill Glackin, shortly after WWII. They shared an apartment in post graduate days at University of California, Berkeley. Glackin, a drama/music critic for the *Sacramento Bee* for over 25 years, was runner up for a Pulitzer Prize.
*Credit: Paul Reese Collection*

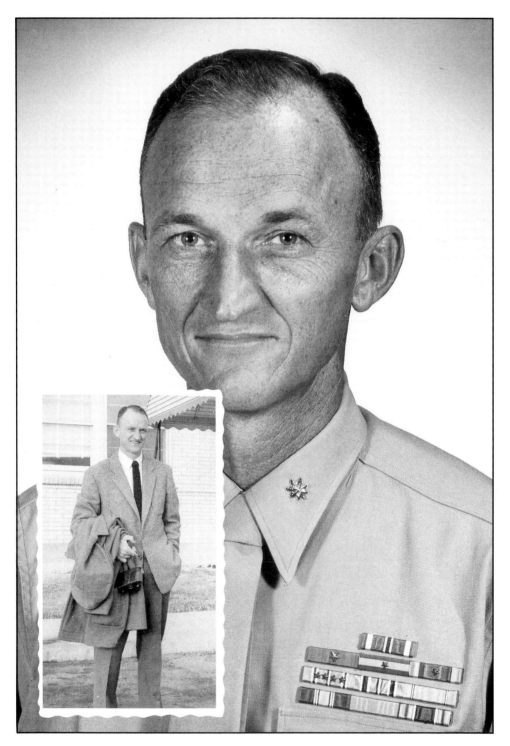

Paul Reese, 1961, when he commanded the 3rd Bn, 4th Marines in Kaneohe, Oahu, and (inset) Paul, 1960 (age 43), as a lieutenant colonel and associate professor of naval science, University of Missouri.
*Credit: Paul Reese Collection*

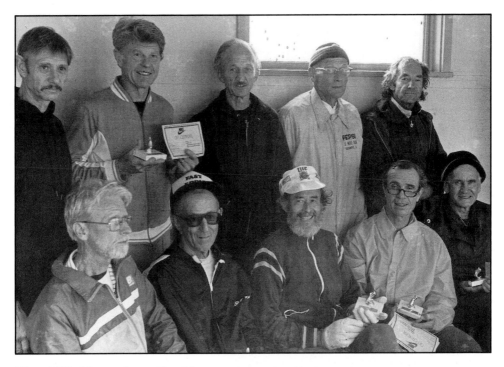

(Above) World record age 60+, 24-hour relay team (209 miles, 1,581 yards, 1 ft., 1 in.). Front row, Harry Harder, Eddie Lewin, Bob Page, Ralph Paffenbarger, George Billingsley. Back row: Frank Grey, John Gilkey, Paul Reese, Ray Mahannah, Don Lundberg.
*Credit: Paul Reese Collection*

(Right) Elaine and Paul Reese when they were directors of the Pepsi 20 Mile Run.
*Credit: Paul Reese Collection*

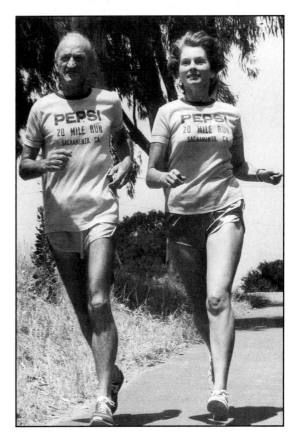

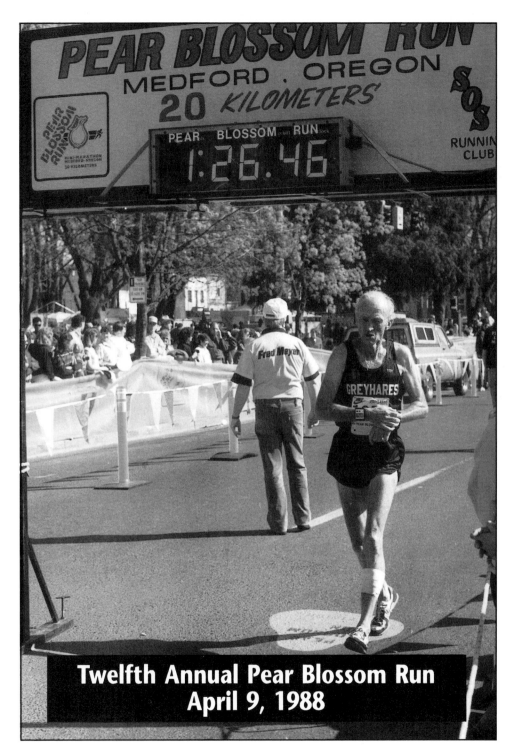

Paul Reese setting national age-70 record for 20K at Pear Blossom Run, Medford, OR, 1988.
*Credit: Paul Reese Collection*

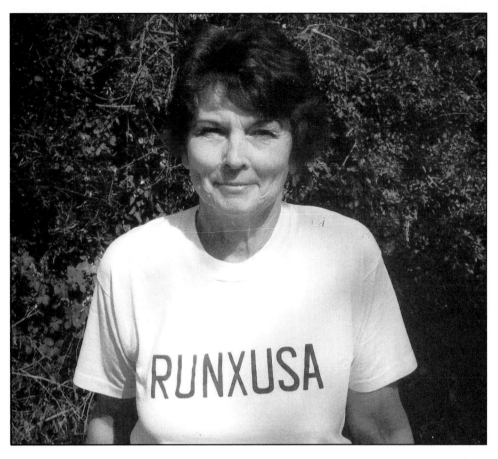

Elaine Reese; (bottom) Elaine's rewards for pit crewing on RUNXUSA, Rebel and Brudder. *Credit: Paul Reese Collection*

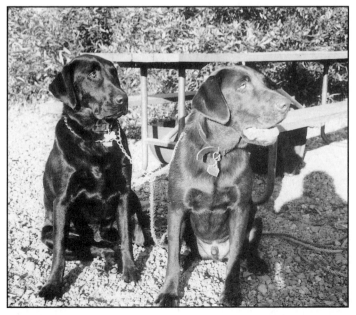

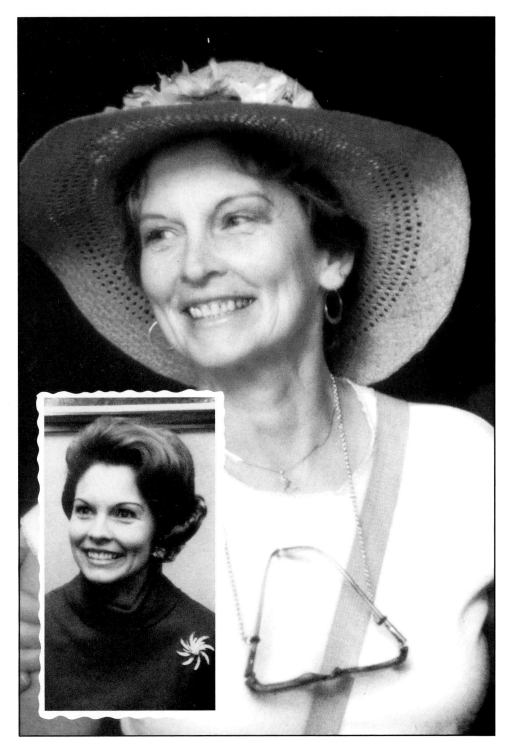

Elaine enjoying Kauai in Hawaii; (inset) Elaine about the time she and Paul started dating.
*Credit: Paul Reese Collection*

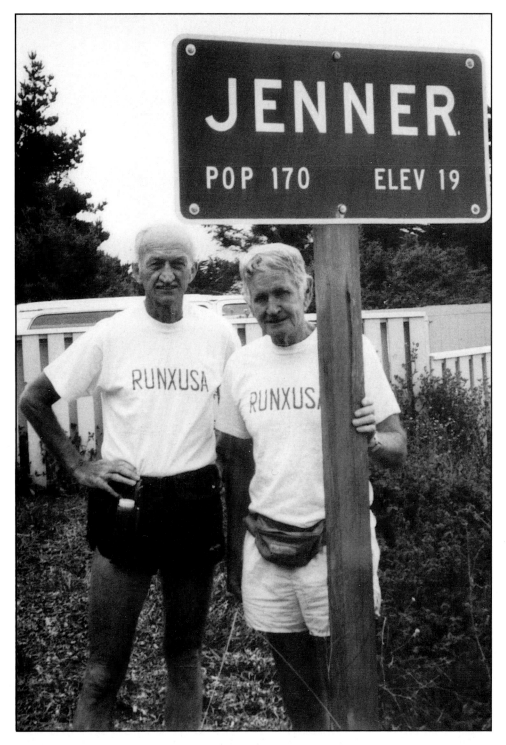

Near start of RUNXUSA, Paul Reese and George Billingsley at town of Jenner, 1990.
*Credit: Paul Reese Collection*

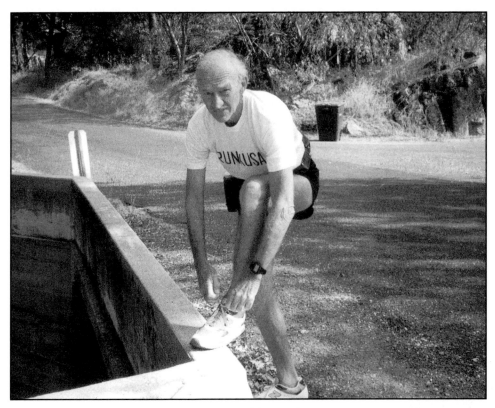

Paul Reese on the road in California (top and bottom).
*Credit: Paul Reese Collection*

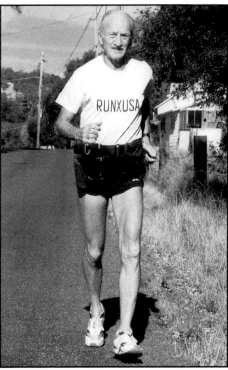

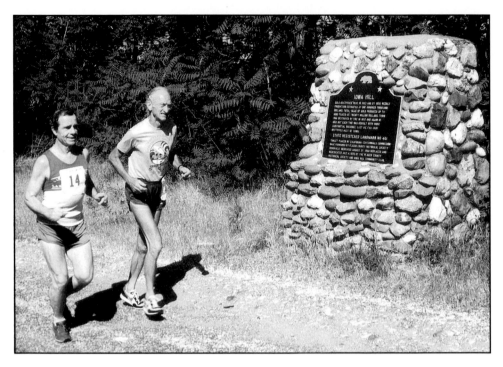

Ralph Paffenbarger and Paul Reese on a Slice 100K Run; (bottom) Elaine Reese hands
Paul a drink.
*Credit: Paul Reese Collection*

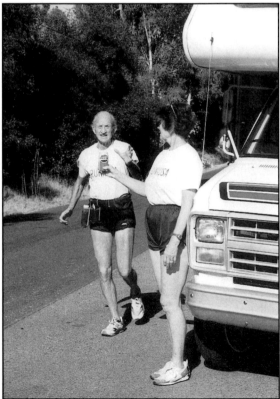

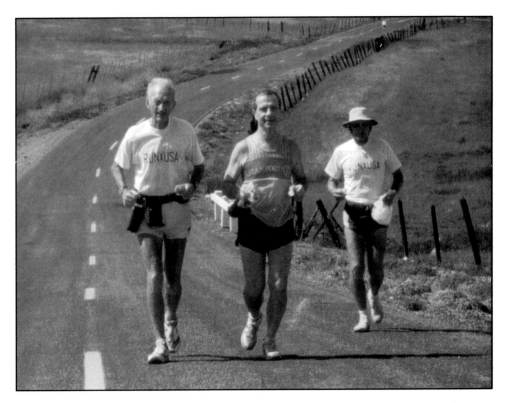

Paul Reese, Ralph Paffenbarger, and George Billingsley on Slice 100K Run, part of RUNXUSA; (bottom) Paul on the road in California.
*Credit: Paul Reese Collection*

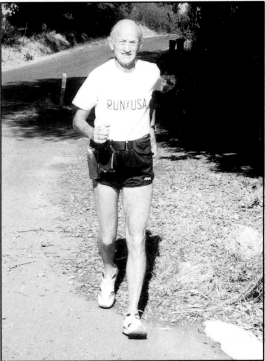

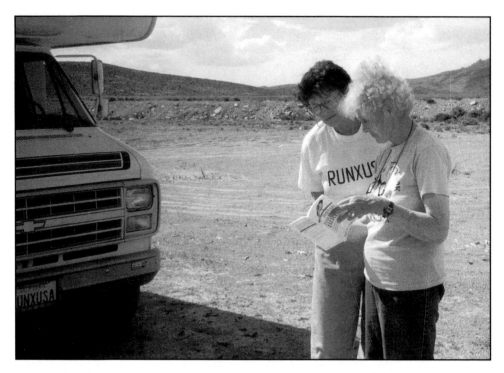

On the Nevada desert, Elaine Reese, left, checks routing with Georgia Billingsley; (bottom) Paul entering Colorado on abandoned Hwy 50.
*Credit: Paul Reese Collection*

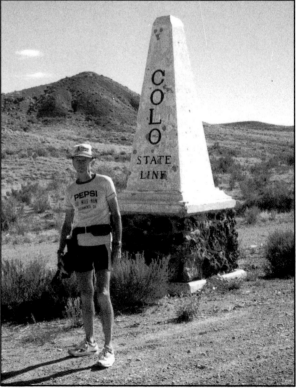

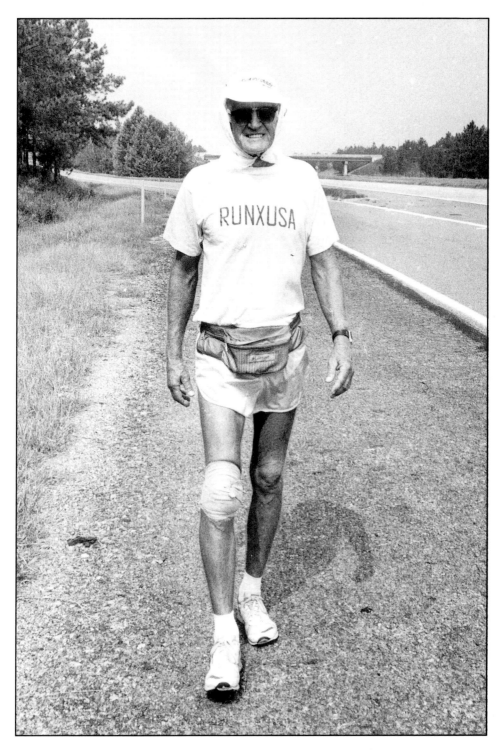

George on the road in Georgia.
*Credit: Paul Reese Collection*

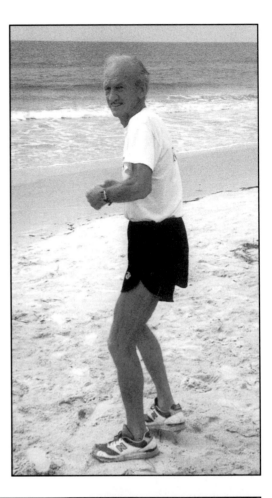

At the finish, Atlantic Ocean,
Hilton Head Island, SC;
(bottom) After finishing in SC,
Elaine and Paul Reese detour to
Miami for a cruise and the easy life.
*Credit: Paul Reese Collection*

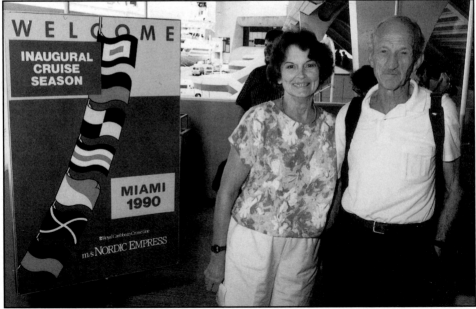

The entire day I ran through the Arkansas River Valley under a clear blue sky and bright sun. There was little wind. East from Sugar City, hundreds of cattle roamed the ranges. As I passed them by, they reacted differently from those I'd encountered earlier in the trek.

Desert cattle were spooked by my presence and ran away wildly. Today's cattle watched me curiously, cautiously, but didn't move. A couple of cows stared at me as if to say, "You damn fool, what are you doing out here so early in your BVDs?"

In a meditative mood this morning, I thought about one of my main purposes in making this run: to awaken people over age 65 to the fact that they have much more physical potential than they realize. But there is some contradiction here, because a person must already be into walking, running, or biking to understand or appreciate the extent and effort of a transcon run.

When I started this run almost 1400 miles ago, I felt confident about cranking out 25 to 26 miles a day. At this point, I still harbor that confidence.

I think the real challenge for someone my age would be 50 kilometers (31.1 miles) per day. I would not want to try that. It would become a physical contest instead of an enjoyable run across the country.

The last two days I've run somewhere between 75 and 80 percent of the time. Attempting that again today, I felt tired at first but was able to stay with it.

A live snake snapped me out of this daydream. Shivers! He lay in a long slit in the blacktop with his head peeking out. That sighting made for a fast leg to the next pit stop!

Soon afterward, a battalion of grasshoppers swarmed nearby. Birds clogged the highway to feed on the grasshoppers. At the same time, horseflies tried to feed on me. I moved fast enough to discourage the flies from landing on me. This resulted in a further drain of energy, already in short supply thanks to Mr. Snake.

We finished at a nondescript spot on the road, then drove to Haswell for overnighting. There are no RV parks within 30 or more miles of here.

Luckily, we located a shady spot in the city park. But the temperature remains uncomfortably hot tonight.

**DAY 56.** A chorus of birds awoke us in the Haswell City Park at 4:10 a.m. Not a day goes by but that I thank God that I am able to do this run.

As I hit the road and began to shake the cobwebs, I thought

of an appropriate phrase I've never used before. Running and walking are brain stimulators.

Guess that's one of the reasons I don't like calisthenics. They don't lend themselves to meditation.

All along Highway 96, we have seen as many abandoned farmhouses as we have active ones. A reflection of the changing scene in America.

Entering Haswell, I found it similar to Sugar City. Both are towns whose time has come and gone, their main streets a series of decaying edifices that give testimony to what the towns once were.

Sugar City is a defunct sugar beet refinery site. Whatever sustained Haswell, I could not determine. Haswell has one active business: a gas station on its east edge. Elaine discovered it and filled the propane tank on the motor home.

When we went through Sugar City a couple of days ago, a tragic event had happened. Two boys, one 12 and one 11, were riding their bikes out of town near a lake. They happened upon a 15-year-old who was tending sheep while armed with a 30-caliber rifle.

That boy delivered an ultimatum to the 12-year-old: "Kiss my toes within five minutes, or I will kill you." When the younger boy refused, the 15-year-old shot him, fatally.

Since arriving in Colorado, we've been able to get a newspaper every day—something we couldn't do in the desert. I read where a kayaker and a rafter were killed a couple of days ago in a boating accident on the Arkansas River.

Recently, we've been reading about the flag burning, which stands as just another example of the deterioration of patriotism in America. Sure, the flag burners are deplorable. But I'm more disappointed by all those citizens who stand idly by and watch rather than thromp the burners.

On Highway 96—like other highways we've traveled in Colorado, Utah, and Nevada—every mile is marked with a green sign. Obviously, the markers make excellent checkpoints.

What we don't know is where does the numbering begin. With a county line, with a state boundary, or what?

As an example of how rummy a runner can get on long treks, I started at milepost 137. Approaching marker 155, I wasn't quite sure whether this was mile 15 or 18. Figuring the answer was almost a matter of higher mathematics.

An uneventful day through the Arkansas River Valley—all under clear skies and through an agricultural setting—came to an end near Eads.

Despite its population of only 878, Eads seems big to us. It has a grocery store, two convenience stores, a bar, two motels, laundromat, county museum, high school, Chamber of Commerce, two liquor stores, a drive-in restaurant, a couple of gas stations—and even RV hookups.

Our first stop was the post office to see if any mail had come for us there. We learned that the post office closed from noon to two P.M. What other business could survive with a two-hour lunch break?

Eads disappointed us in other ways. A motel advertised RV hookups, but they offered no showers and the wrong type of electricity to operate our air conditioner. We stayed anyway, to avoid a 17-mile round trip to the next RV facility.

Elaine and I have acquired a taste for non-alcoholic beer. We tried to find some in the town's two grocery stores and two liquor stores, but came away empty-handed.

Elaine wanted to live it up a bit tonight, which meant walking the three blocks to a nearby highway cafe. Success at last! The chicken fried steak at the Country Kitchen tasted just like what my Aunt Agnes used to cook when I visited my Uncle Paul's ranch.

**DAY 57.** To start this morning, we had to backtrack two miles west from Eads. Elaine spotted a laundromat as we were leaving town, and I later saw her wildly spending quarters there.

The Saturday morning tranquility of the country road was shattered as 15 cattle trucks passed me within a handful of minutes, racing east. The odor from one cattle truck is staggering. Let me tell you, from 15, the effect is overwhelming.

Yesterday's *Pueblo Chieftain* newspaper carried a picture of the typical mountain lion that is roaming the Colorado mountains. Had I seen one of those when I was solo on the roads there, I probably would have suffered cardiac arrest. They look lean, mean, and—above all—hungry.

Towns along today's route showed more of the decay that is typical of this area. Chivington once had a gas station, a grocery store and a two-story brick schoolhouse—all now crumbling. Now the town houses a few trailer homes and two ranch houses.

I learned the town was named for a guy who led a white militia raid that massacred 197 Indians, an act which Congress later deplored. Why have the local folks let the name Chivington stand?

Next came the hamlet of Brandon, which would be better called "Grainville" since it consists of 50 or so grain silos and a huge grain elevator. I saw only four homes and no other businesses.

Things livened up at 22 miles when I encountered Dr. Dan Dracman, of Johns Hopkins University, and his wife. They told me they're biking to Seattle along the Bike Centennial route.

The Dracmans are approaching the trip at a leisurely (for bicycles) 65 miles per day with a van in support. They took pictures of me before we pushed off in our separate directions.

At my last pit stop, I had to take a Pepsi and a Mars candy bar to summon the energy for the final 2-1/2 miles. That wholesome diet did the trick.

The last three days were uppers. I ran well and energetically. But today was somewhat of a downer. Can't pinpoint the reason. Maybe I'm a bit tired, or maybe the scenery has become too repetitious.

Once again, we enjoyed our back-country road, the courteous drivers and the slow pace of life here. But spectacular scenery we didn't have.

East of Eads, much of the land is open range, semi-desert in appearance. Anytime during this day, I could look in a 360-degree circle and see only open space—not a sign of a mountain anywhere.

I might have felt more energetic if I'd known that an RV park with showers and hookups awaited us at the end of the day. The camping books listed none within miles. This was a deficiency in my route planning. I should have checked more carefully for accommodations along the way and maybe re-routed to find better overnight locations.

Surprisingly, we found in Sheridan Lake a cafe that also has RV hookups. This combination was a first for us.

Okay, so the place doesn't offer showers. But bless the air conditioning that let us sit in a motor home in the direct sun and not feel the 90-degree heat outside.

To show our appreciation—and not to heat up the motor home by cooking—we ate in the adjacent Wheatland Cafe. We're always on the lookout for reasons to celebrate. This time it was tomorrow's exit from Colorado and entrance into Kansas.

# E S S A Y

## *The Competitor*
### by Jim O'Neil

*(Jim is the only athlete to participate in every U.S. Masters Track and Field Championships since this meet began in 1968. He has also run in all nine World Veterans Championships. He has medaled in most of these meets. — Paul Reese.)*

Even before I knew him personally, Paul Reese was a hero of mine. When I was a novice masters runner at age 42, it was Paul whom I called to get some badly needed advice to help me get through my first marathon.

My most lasting impression of Paul is watching him compete in the 1972 U.S. Masters Track and Field Championships, where I was an also-ran in the 45–49 division. Competing in the 55–59 age group, he dominated the field in the 5000, 10,000 and marathon—winning these races on successive days, a feat never duplicated in the Nationals before or since.

I realized that I had potential as a masters runner when I finally beat Paul in a race, passing him on the Golden Gate Bridge during a marathon in San Francisco. After the race, Paul came over to me and said, "Well, I see you're a man of your word."

"What do you mean?" I replied.

"Don't you remember at the Pepsi 20 some time ago when I passed you about mile 18 and you yelled to me, 'That's the last time you'll ever pass me in a race.'"

"Oh yeah, I remember now," I said with a smile.

"It looks like that time has arrived," he said, "and that makes you a man of your word. Seems there's no way to keep up with you damn kids. Just remember, I expect great things from you."

Paul has served as an inspiration in my running, and he remains my friend as well as my hero. He exemplifies everything it takes to be a world-class runner.

# Overview of Kansas

## June 17 to July 6 — 499.6 miles — 1970.7 total

| Day | Overnight | Miles | Notes |
| --- | --- | --- | --- |
| 58 | Tribune | 26.4 | last 11.0 miles in Kansas |
| 59 | Leoti | 26.1 | completed 1500 miles |
| 60 | Lake Scott | 26.5 | |
| 61 | Amy | 26.3 | |
| 62 | near Kalvesta | 26.5 | RUNXUSA two months old |
| 63 | Cimarron | 26.3 | reached halfway point |
| 64 | Dodge City | 26.2 | |
| 65 | Ford | 26.1 | |
| 66 | Greensburg | 26.3 | temperature hit 100 degrees |
| 67 | Coldwater Lake | 26.4 | temperature 101 |
| 68 | Medicine Lodge | 26.2 | temperature 100 |
| 69 | Attica | 26.3 | temperature 103, winds 35-40 |
| 70 | Anthony | 26.1 | temperature 104 |
| 71 | Caldwell | 26.2 | |
| 72 | Arkansas City | 26.1 | |
| 73 | Cedar Vale | 26.3 | |
| 74 | Chautaqua | 26.2 | temperature 103 |
| 75 | Caney | 26.1 | temperature 100 |
| 76 | Coffeyville | 26.2 | temperature 102 |

(first 16.2 miles in Kansas on Day 77)

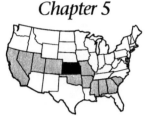

## Chapter 5

# *Will Kansas Ever End?*

Kansas sprawled before us, the widest of our states at a fraction of a mile short of 500. We would spend more time here than in any other state, taking from June 17 through July 6 to make this crossing.

Gone now were the mountains and deserts. Kansas brought the new challenge of crossing the plains where scenery changed little from mile to mile, or even from day to day, and the temperature promised to top 100 degrees for days on end.

I had to fight the feeling of "just put in the miles and get out of here." This wasn't the purpose of RUNXUSA.

**DAY 58.** Wheat fields to the left of me, wheat fields to the right of me. What better way to start the day when we would cross into the state known for its wheat: Kansas.

Early today, I ran back through Sheridan Lake where we'd spent the night. It's ironic that the lake after which the town is named is mostly a dried-up pond. Maybe it overflows with the winter rains.

Speaking of water, it's remarkable that every day or two we've taken it from a different source. As yet, we have suffered no ill effects from this.

I went back to wearing a bandanna today because of my chapped lips. It does protect the lips, but has the disadvantages of impeding breathing and making drinking awkward.

For the past 10 years, ever since Dr. Frank Boutin diagnosed my chronic back problem, I've been wearing a sacroiliac belt while running. Until I began this trek, this had been a six-inch belt.

Because of the heavy mileages of the transcon run and the many hills, I had switched to a nine-inch belt for more protection. That has worked well to this point.

But the nine-incher is heavy and hot as it gets soaked with perspiration. Today, on the rationale that we're out of the mountains, I went back to the lighter and more comfortable six-inch belt. I'll monitor the effects for a few days to see if this change is wise.

Sad sight on the road this morning: a dead buck, a two-pointer. How deer can exist out in this open country befuddles me. They have no cover, only the camouflage of the wheat fields and an army of foes, because who, in this neck of the woods, doesn't hunt?

The flies were out drawing blood from sunup on today. At an early pit stop, Elaine said, "I left the motor home to camcord some wheat fields, and the flies attacked me unmercifully."

Quite unsympathetically, I replied, "Welcome to the club!" This wasn't the tea and sympathy she had expected.

We later made quick work of our camcorder shots at the Kansas state border. The flies feasted on both of us.

It turned out that our highway in Kansas also has markers every mile. This time we knew where they started: right at the state line.

The scenery early in Kansas was as we left it in eastern Colorado—miles and miles of wheat fields. Unfortunately, the Kansas road is narrower and shoulderless.

A mile into Kansas, a damn dog jumped a fence and came after me. I had to use all my command presence and half a dozen rocks to deter him.

Soon afterward, 30 steers stared at me from across the highway with no fence between us. The expressions on their faces read, "Ain't seen nuthin' like this before." I sort of wished there were a tree around here in case they became antagonistic.

I can always tell when I'm approaching a small town around here. First, I see the huge, towering grain elevator. Next, I notice a grove of trees, which are a rarity in this area.

We could spot Tribune, tonight's roosting spot, from the end of today's run eight miles from town. The local grocery store was closed this Sunday, but Elaine can shop there tomorrow as we come through.

Tribune wins our award as the most impressive and pleasant town so far on this highway. It is clean, appears well-managed, has several very nice homes and every service we could require—except an RV park.

We settled again for a city park. Who needs air conditioning in a motor home when the temperature is 90 degrees!

I feel a bit guilty about all the fun I had this Father's Day—jogging 26-plus miles under a hot sun and being chewed on by squads of hungry flies, all this amidst the unwavering scenery of wheat fields. Looks like I'll be spending so much time in the Kansas wheat fields that I could be made an honorary member of the 4-H club.

**DAY 59.** I started somewhat tired from having overextended myself yesterday to escape the flies. Today, by way of surrender, I carried windbreaker trousers to don immediately if I came under attack.

On the Nevada and Utah deserts, I had enjoyed seeing the sun come up—not only because it was a beautiful sight, but also because it brought warmth. Here on the plains, though, I am not anxious to see the sun because it ushers in the oppressive heat and it awakens the flies.

Gonna have to write to the governor about this road. It's too narrow, needs a bike lane, and needs repair. Ninety-six in Colorado was better. Hear me, Guv? When two vehicles approach at the same time, a rare happening on this road, the only alternative I have is to jump onto the bug-infested grass. This act does not exactly inspire mirth.

I read in a newspaper a few days ago where the incidence of Lyme disease in Georgia has increased 60 to 80 percent during the past couple of years. Make a note to stay out of the Georgia grass during our 350 or so miles there.

Sights, sounds and smells from the day:

* I go by a farmhouse and I'm wondering, "Any dogs?" In answer, three of them emerge from a garage and run toward me. "Stay!" I yell in my most forceful voice. Hey, it works! They stop and watch me run away.

* I pass through Horace, a hamlet that looks like it was once hit by a tornado and the folks there subsequently neglected to clean it up.

* Two cattle trucks pass, and their trailing odor leaves me gagging. El stinko grando!

* I go by a rendering plant, and the odor is so foul and engulfing that I find myself on the verge of upchucking. Let me put it this way: Compared with a rendering plant, a Kansas cattle truck is perfume!

* The wind, which peaks at about 40 miles an hour, has kept the flies away. Blessed be the wind!

* A bit of rain and hail the last couple of miles. Wind and hail are, we're told, early signs of a tornado.

Finished running, we drove to Leoti. Again, no RV park. But we got permission to occupy a shady spot at the local high school, courtesy of Bob Spiker.

**DAY 60.** The change to Central Time resulted in a pitch-dark start. This reminded me of similar starts, flashlight in hand, on the Nevada and Utah deserts. The difference today was 60-degree weather compared to those freezing desert mornings.

Both Elaine and I felt a bit tired today because we had had a restless night. The heat, for one thing, and a thunder and lightning storm for another.

This was one of those days that supposedly builds character. Left foot was wobbly, my shoes were too small, the road became narrower and the traffic heavier, the temperature was 95 to 100 degrees and the flies were biting with a vengeance.

Who could ask for anything more? Oh, yes, I neglected to mention the tornado warnings. All this made it a bit difficult to remember our theme: ENJOY.

I can now emphatically declare that Cutter's insect repellent and Off are useless against these Kansas flies. It's like trying to use a .22-caliber pistol to stop a tank.

By the end of yesterday's run, I found my feet have swollen so much that my shoes are now a half-size too small. They are beginning to cause pain and could lead to blisters.

I have no immediate way to buy any larger shoes. My only course of action is to cut out the toebox in the present ones and see what happens.

As we approach the halfway mark in this transcon run, it's frightening to think how delicate the balance is between finishing or not. One sudden disaster—an injury, an accident—could abort it.

Back to Highway 96. Folks here were so friendly in waving today that I was required to expend some of my limited energy to return their greetings.

While I was taking a pit stop beside some mailboxes, the mail carrier drove up, saw my RUNXUSA T-shirt, and commented, "RUNXUSA? You're too old to be doing that!" He didn't know it, but he'd uttered fighting words that will carry me another 500 miles.

Funny how things all come together. For several days, I'd

mentioned to Elaine, "I'm craving bacon and eggs for breakfast instead of the usual oatmeal or cream of wheat." I had bacon and eggs this morning.

So what happened at a pit stop a short while later? Elaine parked across from the Prairie Pork Center, where farmers are delivering truckload after truckload of squealing pigs. Need the guy who had bacon for breakfast say more?

We finished another somewhat uneventful day through the Kansas wheat fields, and decided to drive 15 miles to Lake Scott to see some different scenery—and to indulge in an RV hookup and showers at a state park. The park is adequate but considerably below California standards. Leaves me wondering why Kansans are so tolerant of second-rate roads and facilities.

Around dinnertime, a park ranger knocked on our door to alert us to a storm warning. That was an overture to a night of rain, hail, heavy wind, thunder, and spectacular lightning.

**DAY 61.** Trying to avoid the flies on Highway 96, and also to escape the heavy wheat-harvest traffic on that road, we turned south on Highway 83 this morning and followed it for eight miles. I found 83 to be another example of inferior Kansas roads—too narrow and sadly in need of repair.

Even though I ran facing traffic, I couldn't judge whether a car going my way might be passing another. If the driver of the passing car didn't see me in time, that could spell big trouble since there wasn't space on the road for two cars and me.

For approaching cars, I had two alternatives: jump off into the weeds or cross to the other side of the road if no vehicle was approaching there. The past three days, I've run considerable extra mileage just zigzagging across the road— and this is mileage that doesn't count.

After some map study, we daringly turned onto Shallow Water Road for today's remaining miles. Running this deserted gravel backroad was stimulating, not energy draining as on a busy highway.

I'm lucky in that Elaine also prefers these back roads and is willing to explore them even when we have sketchy map information. Lucky, too, that she is so adept at reading maps.

Our whole time on Shallow Water Road, we encountered only six vehicles. Every one of the drivers stopped to ask if we needed help, whereupon we did our RUNXUSA spiel. One seasoned old farmer looked at me as if to say, "You must be crazy!"

The day's critter report:

* One thing for sure about the Kansas we've been in the past few days: if you don't have a dog in the back of your pickup, you're not with the program.

* I passed by four farmhouses and, surprisingly, not a single dog came out to chase me. Maybe all the dogs were out riding in pickups.

* A maternal scene: eight mares and their newly born colts. We stopped to camcord some of this activity.

* This area must be paradise for pheasant hunters. I jumped eight of the birds along Shallow Water Road.

Elaine and I were treated to watching the first stages of a crew harvesting a wheat field. Three threshers, two trucks and a pickup drove into the field, lined up in their harvesting formation, and began the operation. Their teamwork was precise, with no wasted time or motion.

We finished near the wheat-harvest area, then had to migrate to find a spot for overnight parking. Great as the back roads are, they do present a logistical problem: no RV parks are nearby. Obviously, these parks seek the flow of traffic.

We drove to the hamlet of Amy, which consists of four homes, a grain elevator and an abandoned elementary school. We parked under a shade tree near the school, then explained to the school's neighbor what we were doing. He told us to enjoy.

It occurs to me that we're going into our third month, and I've not yet found an easy way to do 26 miles. At the end of each day, I experience varying degrees of tiredness—some days more, some days less—but I'm always tired.

If we can maintain our 26-mile-a-day pace, we stand a good chance of finishing by August 22, which would make the trek four months long. Our original projection was August 31.

I sometimes wonder, had I known beforehand what a big bite I was taking with this transcon run, if I would have opened my mouth in the first place. On the other hand, I am experiencing an undercurrent of enjoyment through all this trek. Besides, hopefully I'm making some sort of a statement about aging and activity.

This brings to mind something that I read last night in Sammy Davis Jr.'s autobiography, *Why Me?* A highly regarded orthopedist is giving Davis advice about his bad hip and says, "You're suffering from dancer's or athlete's degeneration. You've been using your bones and your sockets harder and for more time than they're made to withstand.

"You're taking a 60-year-old hip socket and grinding it hard twice at night. Take a piece of wood and do that for 10 minutes a night for only a year and see what happens."

I wonder what this same orthopedist would have told me had I approached him with my plan to run across the USA at age 73. What would he think of my having been a distance runner for 27 years and having logged more than 103,000 miles?

**DAY 62.** The featured attraction of the day has been the weather. As we drove the nine miles from Amy to start this morning, the elements were with us: lightning to the east and west, some thunder, strong winds, and a sky full of dark clouds.

While at times a deluge appeared inevitable, the rain never came. I ran under an umbrella of ominous clouds all day, and the wind never abated.

I eased cautiously into the day's run, realizing that early morning running, without warmup, invites injuries. This morning, the problem wasn't the left knee that had bugged me yesterday but rather the arthritis in my left foot. It seems that one encumbrance of being an old runner is to always be plagued with some sort of a nagging injury.

Going along, I noticed that a number of farms along Shallow Water Road had oil wells. Little wonder some of the farm buildings reflected prosperity.

In almost three hours on that road, we encountered only one car. But this setting wasn't as restful as yesterday's because of the road's gravel and dirt composition.

With rain threatening, I hustled as fast as I could. Elaine and I worried that if rain soaked the road, the motor home might get mired. Luckily, we reached paved Highway 23 before any rain fell. This road was also lightly traveled, and its blacktop surface was superior to that of Highway 96.

I faced a strong head wind on this new road, but it was more friend than foe. It kept the flies away and had a cooling effect this warm day.

One feature of the quiet roads that Elaine likes is she can escape from the motor home and work in a short jog while waiting for me. When she was jogging on Highway 23, nine drivers stopped to ask if she needed help. Similarly, the first five pickup drivers who passed me asked if I was okay.

Elaine and I are both impressed with the concern of the Kansas folks. We also agree that similar concern on a California state highway would be nothing short of a miracle.

The nearest city was too far from today's finish line to warrant a commute, so an RV park was out of the question. We parked in a rest area when we heard a radio announcement of a tornado alert in Seward County, 57 miles to the south. Our area has thunderstorm warnings. Sounds as if we will be surrounded all evening by entertaining weather. Not much we can do but batten down the hatches—and pray.

Yes, the weather is the featured attraction today. Hopefully, the tornado will play to an empty house tonight.

**DAY 63.** Looking to the east as my day began, I could see a faint pink glow across the horizon which told me the sun was on its way. The wind whistled again, bending the wheat.

I read in yesterday's newspaper that unseasonable hail had ruined a number of wheat crops in this area. Farmers with hail insurance, I learned, can recover expenses.

Traffic was blissfully light again today. Fifteen or 20 minutes often elapsed without a single car passing.

Late in the day's run, I uttered two prayers of thanksgiving: one, that only a half-dozen flies had descended on me, the other, that I didn't have any signals of potential injuries.

Running along, I found myself mulling over a question that Elaine and I had discussed last night: "What do you consider to be the five main accomplishments of your life?"

I had instantly replied that this transcon run, if completed, would be one. Others I'd consider: serving in five major combat operations with sufficient distinction to earn some decorations (despite not being by natural instinct the brave type); attaining the rank of lieutenant colonel in the Marine Corps; raising three children, all college graduates and well-adjusted; graduating from University of California, Berkeley, with honors.

Offhand, Elaine had cited her professional success as an Assistant Superintendent, Business Services, and her raising of three children.

Another day through Kansas wheat fields and some sunflowers. What made the day unusual was that the wind stayed light, the flies were few, the sky was without lightning and thunder and even clouds, and the heat was not oppressive. Can this be Kansas?

We finished just inside the Cimarron city limits. The town's name stirred memories of my youth. I can still remember seeing Richard Dix in the movie of that name at the then-new Fox Theater in Sacramento. A guy has to have been around quite a while to know who Richard Dix was.

Since for three nights we hadn't been near a town with shopping facilities, Elaine hot rodded it to a grocery store. The next move was to determine if there were any RV hookups in Cimarron. The camping book listed none, but three times already we'd found the book wrong.

Again that turned out to be the case. We found a place with water, sewer and 15-amp electricity hookup (good enough for our lights and for charging batteries, but not for air conditioning). No showers here, but that's no problem since the one in the motor home is quite adequate if we have a water hookup.

It appears that excitement is not in tonight's script. Unlike the past three nights, there are no tornado or thunderstorm warnings.

**DAY 64.** What impressed me most about Cimmaron—our starting point this morning—was the extreme number of trees, something we've not been seeing on the Kansas plains. Hundreds of trees loaded with singing birds.

Many houses in this town had bicycles on their front porches, and some cars had their windows down. Imagine the results of that in almost any American city today. It would be a field day for thieves.

I passed the Cimarron Hotel, established in 1886, and wish I'd seen it yesterday when I could have camcorded and toured it. Downtown I went by Clark's Pharmacy, old-fashioned enough to have the type of soda fountain that characterized drugstores of my youth.

A quarter-mile out of Cimarron, I was back into the wheat fields for the rest of the day. Out in these fields, I heard something that sounded like the prop noise of an old airplane.

A local farmer told Elaine these are water pumps for irrigation. They can be heard at least half a mile away. The farmer said, "It's a noise we live with because it brings the water that we need to make a living out here."

A peculiarity of Kansas I'm noticing is that most farmhouses have a basketball hoop nearby. I received a fringe benefit from basketball today.

A German Shepherd headed out from a house to chase me.

The kid who lived there was shooting baskets, and I yelled to him, "Call your dog!" He shouted, "Buck!" and the dog instantly broke off the chase. I thought, "Hey, kid, I'm glad you were out there shooting." I turned to watch him sink four successive shots.

Kids in this rural area learn responsibility early. I see many of them—15, 16, 17—driving trucks and tractors.

Elaine and I have noticed that all the Kansas farmers have a standardized wave as they drive past. Their hand barely leaves the steering wheel as they hoist two fingers, a gesture which expends a modicum of energy.

Elaine has told me, "The Idaho wave is somewhat similar, and it is considered rude not to return the wave." This means that, since the car's windshield and speed reduce visibility, I have to look closely to see if the driver waves. If he does, I cheerfully return the greeting—at considerable expense to my rationed energy system.

It was sheer pleasure to run down the center of Highway 23 this morning. Bad roads, heavy traffic, and miserable weather make me appreciate this tranquility.

This was one of those days, though, when I didn't flow. Instead, I had to force the action. My left knee again telegraphed unhappy signals. It is, I suppose, the weakest link in my running armament.

After a dozen miles on Highway 23, we turned east on a gravel road (marked as Y Road; can't get much more back roady than this). For sure, nobody running across the USA has ever taken this route.

Elaine and I agree that our most enjoyable times are on the back roads where we get a better feel for the area and where we escape the pell-mell of the busy highways. Sort of like when I was in Tokyo and got off the Ginza for a better feel for the city and the country.

Not a single inquiry or offer of help today. Is word getting around, "There's a crazy old man hereabouts on a run across the USA?"

After finishing for the day, we decided to drive to the Water Sports Campground on the outskirts of Dodge City to enjoy showers and air conditioning. It is a pleasant campground on the shores of a recreational lake. After another day on the road, the simple pleasures of a shower and cool air transported us to "Ecstasy Land."

**DAY 65.** I'll let my miniature tape recorder do the work today. Here goes another stream-of-consciousness report of our day, as spoken to the recorder.

After Elaine drops me on Ensign-Ford Road at 5:38 in the morning darkness, there's nothing out here but the birds, the wind and this setting of wheat and corn fields. At the top of a small knoll, I can look to the north and see the lights of Dodge City, 10 miles away.

What's this, a newly-surfaced road in Kansas? Great, but it's still primitively narrow.

Eleven miles down and no distress signals, though my old body is somewhat weary. Don't know how much I've drained out of the energy reservoir. Would delight in a day off. But think it a better physical test to see if a man over 70 can run across the USA without a day's rest.

Lookee here, a sign I've not seen before: "Danger. Buffalo. Private game refuge." I look out into the field and see half a dozen buffalo. Reminds me of the Catalina Island Marathon, where the runners follow a road that passes through a herd of grazing buffalo.

It's Sunday, but these Kansas farmers are busy harvesting their wheat crops. One of them in a pickup pulls up alongside me and figuratively grabs my ear. He wants to know, "How old are you?" and I tell him.

He says, "I was born in 1910." Not a gray hair on his head, and he oozes vitality.

He also tells me about his combine accident which required him to get a prosthetic hip joint which hasn't troubled him in 29 years. Then he gets into a story about his great-grandfather.

"After loading a wagon with flour, bacon, beans and other staples, he took off for the California gold rush, leaving behind his wife and six children. After he crossed the Mississippi River at St. Louis, he was never heard from again."

His grandfather, on the other hand, struck it rich in Kansas. He had accumulated enough money to buy fencing to enclose 10 by 7 miles, which, under the laws of the time, made it his property (Some of this land now belongs to the farmer who's telling me this story.)

I ask him how many acres he now owns. He says, "Twenty-six parcels, after giving 44 to my kids." As he leaves, I'm left wondering, "What in the hell is a parcel?"

For the first time today, I have to get off the road for a vehicle—a combine. These things are so big that they take both lanes of the road and still overhang a bit. If a combine encounters a car, a game of musical chairs ensues until the combine is able to find a spot to edge off the road and turn sideways—after which the waiting car edges by.

I think that the rule on building roads in Kansas is this: if the road will accommodate a combine, it's a super highway.

A woman in a rather large car stops to ask, "Are you just out hiking?" Hell, I'd rather hike on the Matterhorn than on this narrow-gauge road. Politely, good trooper that I am, I brief her on my mission. When I mention my wife being up ahead in a motor home, the woman drives off almost immediately—leaving me to suspect that she had designs on my sexy senior citizen body!

Here's an indicator that I am getting tired or a report to file with the piss/bitch/moan department: the last hour today is miserable. The road belongs to the 1920s or 1930s, I'm constantly jumping to the rough shoulder of the road at the risk of injury, a head wind impedes my progress, the Sunday traffic is bumper-to-bumper, and combines run me far off the road three or four times.

Today's the worst finish I can recall to date. My right groin, left knee, and right hip are all complaining and expressing doubts about being A-okay tomorrow.

What happened to ENJOYING? That will come tomorrow if I can resurrect from today.

**DAY 66.** When I finished yesterday, much of my lower body was about ready to go on strike. Today, all parts were back on the job. Why the transformation, I don't know.

Still, I don't seem to be recovering as well overnight as I was a while back. This morning, for example, the metatarsals in my right foot were rebelling.

What the hell, though. There's always something amiss or close to amiss. Being tired—almost inescapable on this type of run—means being highly susceptible to injury. Part of the trick to avoid debilitating injuries is to keep tuned for distress signals and to honor or respect them.

Good news came early today. A farmer in a pickup pulled alongside me and asked, "Are you another one of those cross-country runners?"

The question startled me. "Another?"

I pleaded guilty. He then said, "The day before yesterday I talked with a guy named Billingsley who went through here."

I calculated from his report that George was approximately 40 miles ahead of us. That figured, since his mainline highway routes were about that much shorter than our back roads.

The farmer then got out of his pickup and, on its dusty hood diagrammed a route to Medicine Lodge. His option put us onto back roads again.

I thanked him for his help. Then Elaine and I—back road demons that we are—gladly followed his routing. We doubted that George and Georgia took this same advice.

Before reaching the sanctuary of the alternate road, I had to brave more of Highway 54. It was the busiest we'd been on for quite a spell.

This highway was newly surfaced blacktop without an inch of paved shoulder. Since there is plenty of space for one, I have a difficult time understanding the mentality that would construct such a rinky-dink highway.

The thought struck me that, during all our days in Kansas, we have not seen a state Highway Patrol officer. It's understandable, though, why one would be reluctant to drive these highways.

When we planned this trip, we had no apprehensions about Kansas. But this state, with its narrow roads, flies, and erratic weather, has been a problem. Its redeeming feature has been the fine folks we have met.

By the time I finished, the temperature topped 100 degrees. Elaine and I retreated nine miles to Greensburg for the creature comforts, particularly air conditioning, of an RV park.

Besides, it was time to restock groceries, propane, and gas. In Greensburg—which boasted the world's largest hand-dug well—I finally saw a piece of honest advertising. Dillon's market claimed, "The best groceries in Greensburg."

Couldn't argue with that. It was the ONLY grocery market in town.

**DAY 67.** The weather at today's start reminded me of the Honolulu Marathon: warm, balmy air in which running shorts and T-shirt feel comfortable.

Radio weather reports said the temperature would be over 100 degrees. I wondered, "Why wasn't I out on the road at four a.m. instead of 5:37?"

My preoccupation with time is so great that I'm still wearing two wristwatches. The one on my right wrist simply gives the time of day. I use the one on my left wrist as a stopwatch to time myself between pit stops.

True, I could use the same watch for both purposes, but I don't want to bother changing modes frequently. My two watches give me instant time of day and an instant reading of how long it has been since I left the motor home.

Every time I go by a Kansas farmhouse, I move to the opposite side of the road to give more reaction time in case a dog comes charging out. Dogs come out friend and foe, but I worry about both types. The foes might do nasty things to my flesh, and the friendlies might get hit by a speeding car.

Observations about Kansas farmers: don't try to sell them a small car. The cars I see parked in front of these farmhouses are all big—Cadillacs, Chrysler New Yorkers, Olds 98s, Ford LTDs.

Another observation, with which Elaine agrees: About one-third of the cars are driven by women alone, with nobody else in the car. The sociological significance of that escapes me.

About halfway through today's run, a farmer in a pickup stopped and asked with a concerned look, "Do you know that the next town is 41 miles away?" He relaxed when I told him Elaine was ahead in a motor home to support me.

My injury of the day was in the metatarsal area of the left foot. I'd be running along fine, then suddenly a twitch, a pain, and the foot buckled. I'd back off, walk, and then resume running. This process was repeated several times. I don't have to be a physiologist to know that this injury is a fallout from overuse. What the hell, though, this will cease after another 1,400 miles!

As I go along, I'm sort of in a crossroads between what runners call "associating" and "disassociating." I need to associate—pay strict attention to what I'm feeling at the moment—to catch signals of potential injuries and to practice preventive medicine or therapy.

Yet I need to disassociate—that is, get my mind off running—to make the effort easier. Disassociating is forgetting all about running and, as one example, thinking back to my days at the University of California in Berkeley.

That was Depression time when every penny counted. One reason I chose UC was that the yearly tuition was only $52. Joe Quintana and I shared an "apartment" consisting of a bedroom and kitchen (the common toilet was off the hallway, and we took showers in the university gym). Our monthly rent was $16.

I still remember my typical Monday through Friday lunch: a peanut butter sandwich on French bread. In those days, a loaf of this bread cost 10 cents, the same price as a jar of peanut butter.

Disassociating, I even played around with some doggerel and came up with this:

"I hear the moans from weary old bones.
Tired old tendons need mending.
Some bones seem close to breaking.
But one thing for sure, I can say,
As we do our 26-mile day,
That we're gonna stay in motion
And put our feet in the Atlantic Ocean."

The temperature when we finished was 101 degrees. Percy Cerutty, a great Australian running coach, used to teach, "Run until you're exhausted. Then you are ready to begin meaningful training." By that standard, I'm ready.

**DAY 68.** It was a pleasure, on two counts, to return to Highway 160 this morning. First, we knew the traffic would be light, and, second, today would bring us into Medicine Lodge, at whose post office I'm supposed to pick up some new shoes that fit.

My feet have swelled to the point where my present shoes are too small. For 10 days, I've been running in shoes with the big toe cut out.

I loved today's traffic—or lack of same. We saw only six cars in the first two hours and none for stretches as long as five miles.

Elaine and I agree on these impressions of the Kansas vehicle code: Farm equipment takes precedence over cars and pedestrians; anybody can adorn his vehicle with a flashing yellow light and use it at will; as long as a truck carries an "oversize" sign, it can be even wider than the road lane; as far as weight limit is concerned, any truck that does not sink through the pavement is okay.

Luckily, no injury signals appeared today. I had a good flow going, especially on the downhills. This was my easiest day in quite a spell. Mind you, I did not say an "easy day." None is. But I wish I knew the reason for it being one of the easiest.

Blushingly, I admit to indulging in more nonsense today.

Trying to disassociate—to get my mind off running—I spent a good deal of time polishing the doggerel that started yesterday. The result:

"You can hear the moans
From my weary bones.
Every muscle is so sore
It's screaming, 'No more.'

"And every single tendon
Stands in need of mending.
Yes, old bones are aching
To the point of breaking.

"Add to that, my ancient back
Is completely out of whack.
As my legs hit the ground
And go pound, pound, pound.

"Each pound thrice my body weight,
Is a happening that they hate.
Yet I remain like a kid with a toy
Because, throughout, I do enjoy."

Today began on a pleasant note—with the empty road and absence of injuries. It also ended on a pleasant note.

A quarter-mile from where Elaine was waiting at the finish, a German Shepherd emerged from a farmhouse, exuding signs of friendliness. I greeted him and we frolicked a couple of minutes, after which he retreated home. My kind of dog.

At the finish, Elaine had a root beer float for each of us. That's living!

We drove into Medicine Lodge and got bad news. My shoes hadn't arrived at the post office. We'll have to try again tomorrow.

Elaine announced that tonight the schedule calls for dinner out. I had suspected that and was prepared.

The natives whom I asked reported that the Hereford House is "the best restaurant in town." We'll see.

**DAY 69.** An unusually early start this morning, 4:59 a.m., because the temperature was 74 degrees and not conducive to sleeping. A weather report from Wichita said the heat index today would reach 110. Gotta find out exactly what's meant by "heat index."

A report on last night's dinner at the Hereford House: It's hard to beat this small-town Kansas restaurant for price. For $4.75, we had a salad bar, chicken fried steak, mashed potatoes and gravy, and toast. My iced tea, cheerfully refilled, was 40 cents.

Elaine went to check on my shoes at the Medicine Lodge Post Office this morning and returned with the disappointing news that they hadn't arrived. She left instructions for them to be forwarded to Coffeyville. Meanwhile, I trudge on in a pair that's too small and with the toe area cut out (Hey, my big toes should get a suntan!). Could be worse; I could be barefoot.

Medicine Lodge is an interesting little town. It was the home of Carrie Nation, and that home is preserved as a museum. We visited it yesterday. Like all the other small Kansas towns, Medicine Lodge has a city park. This one is large, considering the population, and exceptionally well-maintained. There is also an attractive golf course on the east edge of town.

If I had to use only one word to describe these small Kansas towns, it would be "character." These towns seem to reflect the rugged individualism of the Kansans.

After leaving Medicine Lodge, I stopped to read an historical marker that told of the Kiowa, the Comanche, the Arapaho, and the Cheyenne Indians signing a peace treaty here with the federal government in 1867. Fifteen thousand Indians camped here during the council, and 500 soldiers escorted the U.S. Commissioners. (I wondered who was running the local McDonald's at the time to feed all these people.)

The treaty, while not guaranteeing peace, did clear the way for the railroad and eventual settlement. Eastern newspapers were interested enough to send correspondents to cover the event. One reporter was Henry Stanley, who later found Livingston in Africa.

Back to running. Two things have remained constant all day: the unvarying scenery (flatlands, wheat fields and cattle-grazing lands) and my lack of energy. I didn't have the juice today.

Some days—and this is one of them—the 26 miles seem eternal. The only recourse is to not think in terms of the whole 26, but to work from one pit stop to the next. Forward progress. In time, the miles do accumulate. You're glad then that you did hang in there, and you hope that tomorrow will be better.

On a long trek like this, a runner has to take the ups and downs, and work around them. But the psyche should remain constant. By that, I mean upbeat.

Today's traffic flowed heavier than yesterday's, but it was still quite tolerable. As I reached the town of Sharon, I discovered my first miracle in Kansas: a paved shoulder on a Kansas state highway. Surprisingly, this runable shoulder extended for 10 miles. Kansas should decorate the imaginative soul who planned this road.

The first sign I saw while passing through Attica was that the local Bulldogs had won the state football championship in 1988. This town was a welcome sight because it marked our finish line.

'Tis a day I'm glad to see wind down. The 35- to 40-mile-per-hour crosswinds, along with the 100-plus temperatures (103 at the finish), zapped me.

It's another one of those nights when we go to bed hoping tomorrow will be better. Amend that: PRAYING tomorrow will be better.

**DAY 70.** I performed some delicate surgery last night and this morning. What I did was take a new pair of New Balance 840 shoes (we're talking $79.95 retail) and cut the toebox out of each shoe, similar to the way I had done with an old pair.

The old ones had lost their cushioning protection after 545 miles of life. So to protect the weary warrior at any cost, I performed the surgery.

The trick of the surgery is to allow the big toe and the one next to it to expand and not jam against the shoe's toebox to create blisters. The operation appears to be a success. The shoes feel fine.

Amazing how much more I feel like running with the cushion in these shoes as compared with the lack of desire yesterday in broken-down shoes. However, there is now the chance of my exposed toes getting cut by glass, tin, or rocks when I'm forced off the highway into the weeds. *C'est le guerre!*

A course record of a type today: shortly after I started, seven dogs came out from a small farm across the road. They barked, then nudged under the fence and came out to the edge of the highway.

But, on my command, they stopped. Prayers answered.

However, my prayers for friendly winds went unanswered. I fought 35- to 40-mile-per-hour head winds for many miles.

I'm learning that it is foolhardy to try to run hard against that wind force. It wastes energy.

Wind is an element we did not anticipate when planning this trip, yet it has been an almost constant companion. I'd estimate that 10 percent of the time it's been a tail wind, 35 percent a head wind, and 55 percent a crosswind.

Highway 14, where we spent much of today, is another typical Kansas state road. As Ronald Reagan said in another context, "If you've seen one, you've seen 'em all!" Combine-wide, no shoulder, and in need of some repair.

I passed Chaparral High School and wished I had time to study the design. It looked imaginative (sort of like the Taj Mahal) and functional compared to the structures we've been seeing.

Right on the edge of the school property was a billboard advertising a funeral home in Anthony. If I'd seen this sign in the afternoon yesterday, while finishing 26 miles in 103-degree heat, I might have considered applying for admission.

As I approached the town of Anthony, I saw a functioning drive-in theater. Since it doesn't get dark hereabouts until about 9:30 these summer nights, I wondered how late these folks stay up when they attend these movies.

Before catching up with me in Anthony, Elaine took a detour to the town of Harper to buy an electrical adapter to give us more flexibility with the motor home. This adapter will allow us to plug into a 50-amp box, a capability we did not have before. Many RV parks have only this type of connection while our system is 30 amps.

In Anthony, Elaine found the local yardage shop (the first in many a town) and stopped to buy some material to make a dress, which should keep her occupied for a while. She also gave the local laundromat some business.

Before leaving town, we stumbled across an article about George Billingsley in the local newspaper. Seems he had come through Anthony last Monday and made the local press.

People have been asking me, "Are you the guy in the paper?" Now I know what they are talking about. My standard answer is, "No, he's a 68-year-old kid, and I'm 73."

Well, as I wind up the day, I'd say it was not difficult, but it was laborious. What day isn't?

Most of these days, Elaine serves me a root beer float when I finish. Lawdy me, at that moment I do believe I see the pearly gates!

**DAY 71.** Elaine and I exercised exceptional character this morning by getting up at 3:45 a.m. for our long drive to the starting area. We were on the road, running, at 4:55 a.m.

It was pitch dark at the start but a warm 72 degrees. All I needed was a sarong, and I'd have been in Polynesia.

Early today, the old Irving Berlin tune, "I Hate to Get Up in the Morning" ran through my head. Don't think I've mentioned this before, but the most sleep I get any night is nine hours. I'm not sure that is sufficient for recuperability, especially at my age.

When we first came into Kansas, I felt sorry for the farmers I saw working the fields in this heat. Then I learned that much of the farm equipment nowadays is air-conditioned. Hell, they're more comfortable than I am out on the road.

As I left Highway 44 for 49, I passed a monument commemorating Jesse Chisholm and the Chisholm Trail. Ah yes, courtesy of John Wayne, I remember it well.

A lady driver stopped to report that she saw George walking through here four days ago. She wanted to know, "Are you headed for Atlanta, too?" Where she got Atlanta as our destination is a mystery to me.

Then she asked an unusual question: "Are you going to write a book?"

I told her, "I'm keeping a log, but the publishing market is not ripe for a running book. Besides, my writing is not that good."

"Are you sure you won't be coming out with a book?" she asked.

"I doubt it," I answered, "But I sure would like to be wrong."

Now here's a corker: A woman driving a Cadillac with Oklahoma plates stopped and asked me if the motor home a ways back was mine. When I said it was, she wanted to know, "Are you interested in selling it?"

I explained to her that it is our lifeline to the Atlantic. Well, not quite in those words, but I did tell her it most definitely was not for sale.

This was my day for human contact. Four Kansas farmers asked if I needed help, and even the driver of a semi stopped. Lord, I must have looked awful!

We chose Caldwell for our overnighting spot, partly because Elaine identifies with the name. She was born and raised in Caldwell, Idaho.

There are many beautiful, shady trees in Caldwell. I could easily lie down under any one and take a blissful nap. On the outskirts of Caldwell is a motel which carries a sign I've never seen on a motel marquee, "Storm shelter"—which tells a story about the local weather.

Finishing and searching for an RV hookup, we ran into a unique situation. We were referred to a private home where, for $10, the owner hooked us up with 50-watt power (lucky we bought that converter) and water. Always something different.

**DAY 72.** This dark morning, we crossed the Chikaskia River for the third time in two days. I wonder how many times Chisholm crossed it, and if Chikaskia is an Indian word does it mean, "Oh, river to be crossed many times?"

This is Sunday, and in the first two hours the traffic quadrupled that of all day yesterday. Ask me not why. For sure, they couldn't all be going to church.

My left knee was rebellious by the time I finished last night, and it wasn't too cooperative today. All injuries are scary, but knees especially so. Muscles and tendons can be taped, but not knees.

A new problem flared up today. I had trouble with equilibrium. Right after I stopped running and walked a few steps, I felt as if I might fall—or as if I was sliding or walking on ice. I had an overture of this yesterday, but it was short-lived.

For about a week last January, I had had similar symptoms. The M.D. said then, "If the symptoms persist over a week, I will run some tests." They didn't, and he didn't. Now it is a somewhat frightening experience to feel I am sliding into approaching cars.

These symptoms were with me for a couple of hours this morning. Then I drank a couple of Pepsis and was okay in the afternoon. I am wondering if sugar intake is helpful.

Adding to the problem was beastly Highway 166. Its surface was concrete, and every foot or so there was a slit across the road.

These slits make it hard to keep from stumbling. And on this washboard surface, any car sounded like a freight train and could be heard from a mile away.

Along this infernal road, I spotted three rabbits romping in the grass. Quietly, I tiptoed over there and saw one of them, 10 feet away, hugging the ground in an attempt to hide. Trying not to frighten him, I returned to the road.

Speaking of being frightened, it was somewhat startling each time a car sped by me because of the racket it made on this road. Unfortunately, there was a heavy parade of cars in the direction of Ark City (the natives' name for Arkansas City).

This was another one of those days when one-third of the drivers approaching me had the entire road to themselves but failed to give me any space. I again wondered if this results from a lack of brains or a lack of courtesy.

One bad habit (it could be fatal) I have when I am tired is that I get ticked off and hold my ground. This leaves the driver with the alternatives of hitting me or of moving over.

Tired as I am, I almost always feel more buoyant on the last leg of the day. This probably comes from the satisfaction of having completed another day. Also there's the comforting thought that once I finish, the creature comforts of the motor home await.

As I finish each day, climb into the motor home, and park my fanny on the soft seat, it's restful. Peacefully so.

We end this day having accumulated 1,850 miles. This signals that I must get busy on the 2,000-mile report that we will send to people who asked to be kept informed of our progress.

Also much on my mind is that we will probably have to change some of our routing. Elaine discovered that our Alabama pre-planned route is all red-line (meaning major) highways, and that is something we don't want. We are also giving thought to finishing in Charleston, South Carolina, instead of near Savannah, Georgia.

**DAY 73.** On our way out of Arkansas City this morning, we stopped at a 24-hour grocery store. Elaine tried to buy some non-alcoholic beer (less than 0.5 percent alcohol), but the clerk said, "We can't sell it before six a.m. because of its alcohol content."

But he could sell us all the vanilla extract (35 percent alcohol) or lemon extract (84 percent alcohol) we wanted. Now how's that for a legal snafu?

We were overwhelmed with the size of Arkansas City (population 13,201) after back roading through small towns for so long. Big as it is, though, it does not have an American Automobile Association (AAA) office, I found out yesterday while trying to get some maps.

Nowhere in town could we buy a map of South Carolina. No one here seems to think beyond Kansas, Nebraska and Oklahoma.

Later as I trekked east, Elaine retreated to Arkansas City to pick up mail at the post office. She returned with a letter from her daughter (my step-daughter) Kathy, which was a morale raiser for her.

East of town, I caught sight of a mansion—three stories, brick and almost the size of the White House. The neatly manicured front lawn was a half-mile long and 200 yards wide, and edged on three sides by rows of trees. This occupant must own the oil refinery—or the state.

Highway 166 out of Arkansas City was not a happy trail. It was chipped gravel, narrow gauge with shoulder grass a foot or so high.

The road evolved into a roller-coaster: uphill and downhill all day. In our pre-planning for this run, I had conceived of Kansas as flat. How often it has shown me otherwise.

A persistent problem all day was a task force of gravel trucks—10 or so—at work along our route. Between them and other traffic, I must have crossed the road to avoid vehicles or jumped into the shoulder grass a hundred times. A discouraging waste of energy. But again, who said this would be a picnic?

There was one exceptional scene today, happening just after I crossed Grouse Creek (which appeared to be bigger than many rivers). I came upon a little valley green with alfalfa and ringed with small hills. It was a postcard scene.

When I went by Lake Crowley today and the temperature was 100 degrees, I was reminded of Tarzan Brown. He was leading the Boston Marathon on a hot day about 60 years ago, saw a lake on the way, impetuously stopped off for a swim and as a result of this sojourn lost the race.

The T-shirt I wear reads, "RUNXUSA." Were Elaine and I to redesign the shirt, it would read, "No Problem. On a RUNXUSA."

Why so? Well, 13 people stopped today to ask if I had a problem. Could it have been the heat or my looking like such a sad sack?

I did feel a bit wrung out from the weather. But I'm glad to have survived the entire day with only a slight equilibrium problem, just a touch of imbalance a couple of times early in the morning.

Being wrung out, I reflect on how soothing it is to plop into bed at the end of each day. Three times in my life I have yearned for sleep—first in college, next in combat, and now with this run.

**DAY 74.** We were on the road at 4:50 a.m. after a pleasant night in the Cedar Vale City Park. But even at this early hour, I couldn't beat the traffic. It was like 42nd and Broadway out there—20 vehicles in the first hour compared to the usual one or two.

Shortly east of Cedar Vale, the tone was set for the kind of road and scenery we would confront all day. This was cattle grazing country with small rolling hills. Nowhere was the road level. It dipped into a gully, climbed out, dipped again, ad infinitum. These gullies were risky to run because the drivers weren't aware I was there until they were upon me. The condition for running here is always Red Alert.

The major topic with Elaine and me today was whether or not to change our finish from Savannah, Georgia, to Charleston, South Carolina. At pit stops, Elaine reported she had re-routed us with a Charleston finish and the mileage was close to what it had been for Savannah.

She is anxious for me to check her figures (mathematically speaking!), which is a task I'll get to right after we finish the 2,000-mile letter.

I have one misgiving about Savannah. We would not actually finish there (the only water being the Savannah River), but we would have to go another 20 miles or so to Tybee Island to reach the Atlantic. Thereafter, anytime we told somebody that we finished at Tybee Island, we would have to follow with an explanation of where and what it is.

Charleston, on the other hand, is well known and sits on the Atlantic. Remember those Confederate cannons booming away at Fort Sumter?

Besides, I harbor fond memories of Charleston. On a visit there in 1963, I met General Mark Clark. He offered me a job at the Citadel where he was superintendent. A good friend, Dennis Nicholson, a Marine compadre who worked at the Citadel as a vice-president, lined up the interview. Much as I would have enjoyed the experience of working for General Clark, and as highly as I regarded the Citadel, I passed up the job to settle in my native state of California.

With this scenario, it now appears that we will finish in Charleston. But that seems far away as I pass through places like Sedan and Chautauqua, Kansas. Sedan's merchants advertised the yellow brick sidewalk which connects their downtown stores. The town houses a large Emmett Kelly museum. Seems he came from this part of the country. In Sedan, I noticed an ice cream store, a candy factory, and a place featuring shaved ice. A town with all that is to be envied!

The living is easy tonight at a full-service RV park in Chautauqua. But I have a lot to think about with the 2,000-mile report to family and interested friends to write and with the rerouting to check.

My decision-making power is wavering at this point in the run. But I have made one firm, irreversible decision. When I get to the Atlantic, I'm not turning around and running back to the Pacific.

**DAY 75.** Bing, bang, boom went the fireworks overnight, reminding us that this is the Fourth of July. It would be just another day on the road for us, and we wondered what kind of traffic the holiday would bring. No trucks, I hoped.

It was so balmy and breezy early this morning that I was reminded of Hawaii. Could almost hear the natives singing "Aloha." I don't think a day has gone by in Kansas when, enjoying the 5:30 start, I haven't wished I'd started at 4:30 a.m.

On the down side, it's becoming evident that I'm not recovering as much overnight as I did a couple of months ago. That's probably because some of these injuries are becoming ingrained, imbedded or whatever.

Some equilibrium problems returned this morning. The left foot seemed to slip or feel like it' was slipping, but the right one was okay.

The problem was only temporary, though, and I didn't experience it at all in the afternoon. To be honest, it's always amazing to me that I can feel as tired and stiff as I do in the morning and then can work through it.

Vehicular traffic did turn out to be heavy. Some towed horse trailers, some boats, some racing cars. To each his own this holiday.

Historic moment: For the first time in 18 days in this state, I saw a Kansas Highway Patrol officer. In fact, we had a pleasant chat. Now why couldn't he have been nearby when some jerk threw a firecracker at me as his car passed by today.

Later in the day, I found three miles of sheer ecstasy on

Highway 166/75. The road was blacktop with a bike lane and a breakdown lane.

The engineer who designed this deserves knighthood. The governor of Kansas should bring all the state highway engineers to this road, then say to them, "See it is possible. Now go, thou, and do likewise."

The most unusual aspect of the day was that not a single person stopped to ask if I had a problem. Was this because I looked vigorous or repulsive?

Preceding me, Elaine had scouted out an RV park in Caney. But we arrived to find that, for some mysterious reason, the equipment there didn't work despite the best efforts of the proprietor.

He then offered us an air-conditioned room with private bath in his bed-and-breakfast establishment. So this is how we wound up staying at a B&B for the first time on this trip—actually, the first time in our lives.

**DAY 76.** Because it was difficult to sleep in the bed-and-breakfast place (the "air conditioning" turned out to be a noisy swamp cooler), we were up at four o'clock and out running by 4:55 a.m. We expected little traffic then.

Wrong! It was almost bumper to bumper, a mystery that will remain unsolved.

This was not too easy a day because we did not sleep well last night. In the hot room, we sweated and dehydrated.

On top of that, I had severe stomach cramps this morning. Could have been from the salad bar or pizza last night.

The big excitement today was that in Coffeyville we would be picking up mail. Elaine would go for it when the post office opened.

One of the problems when approaching a large city—and Coffeyville is large in this part of the country, with 15,000 population—is that we pick up an increased volume of traffic. Then, in the city itself, I have to contend with all the cross streets. Americans, they're all in one helluva hurry.

Elaine returned from her chores with mail, groceries and copies of our 2,000-mile report. But the larger shoes I'd ordered didn't arrive. I stuck with too-small shoes that have the toebox cut out.

Today, in the hot weather, I resorted to a trick that Dr. Ralph Paffenbarger and I have used when running ultramarathon races together. At each pit stop, I soaked my T-shirt in cold water, then donned it when I hit the road.

Speaking of Paff, I have been thinking of him today because my son Mark has relayed information that it is possible Paff may need to have heart surgery.

That's hard for me to understand. Here is a guy who has demonstrated unbelievable endurance in the Lake Tahoe 72 Mile Run, Western States 100-Mile Run, Camellia Festival 100-Mile Run and dozens of other races we've run together.

Until now, I had thought that Paff was indomitable. How fantastically enduring the human body, yet sometimes how frighteningly vulnerable.

Back to today: This was another one of those days when, after finishing, we drove miles for an RV hookup—in this case back to Coffeyville. There, we found, the city park had half a dozen hookups and the price was right—only $3.

Elaine insisted on taking me on a tour of downtown Coffeyville. One landmark was the Dalton Gang museum. We arrived too late to visit the museum, but as we passed by a thought crossed my mind. It's ironic that America has so many outlaw and gangster museums and mementos and so few that recognize law-abiding achievers.

We returned to the RV park only moments before a young woman reporter from the local newspaper arrived to interview Elaine and me.

I asked the reporter, "How did you find out about us and our adventure?" We have never attempted to attract publicity.

She said, "I got a phone call from a friend at the place where your wife made copies."

Mystery solved. We enjoyed a pleasant conversation with this young lady, a product of the Journalism School at the University of Kansas. Gretchen Pippenger produced the first known story about us in almost 2-1/2 months on the road.

# E S S A Y

# *The Companion*
by George Billingsley

*(George and I ran through four western states before we took separate routes in Colorado. More about George in later chapters. — Paul Reese.)*

Observing Paul Reese in action has taught me that, while life might not really begin at 65, it most certainly doesn't need to end at that point. With a little luck, a person doesn't have to stop living a life that is fun and exciting.

Nor do good times have to be restricted to the thrills of a spectator or to fantasies. Believe me, this old Marine knows how to live, and he kissed off 65 many years ago.

In describing aging, it has been said, "The lights go out one at a time." This is probably true. But if so, every time one goes out, Paul screws in a new bulb.

In his combat with Father Time, it's amazing how he keeps winning. Atrophy, the horrible creeping killer, doesn't have a chance.

Paul simply won't stay down. Running-induced injuries may slow him down, but they don't stop him. He will walk if he has to. But so far, he has never permitted anything to make him retire from running—or anything else he wants to do.

One of his finest demonstrations as a stubborn old coot who won't give up was when he was undergoing radiation for prostate cancer (at the tender age of 70). He still ran five miles every day.

There's no doubt that Paul is a runner. He has run more miles and more races (at all distances) and faster than almost anyone close to his age.

Yes, running is a major part of Paul's life. But that isn't all he does.

He romances Elaine. He travels. He gives speeches. He directs races. He corresponds. He writes. He paints his two-story house. And the list goes on.

He also enriches lives other than his own. Delightfully, he has helped make our training (for years we've been running together twice a week) fun and our adventures exciting.

Some people think of the good life as resembling the sand in an hourglass that gradually flows through to the bottom. Some people assume that even as young as 65 the good life is all gone, that there is nothing left to trickle through, that all that remains of the good times are memories.

Paul refuses to think this way. He constantly pours more sand into the top of the glass. He persists in doing what restores his capacity for continuing the good life.

# Overview of Oklahoma

## July 6 to July 8, 1990 — 44.0 miles — 2014.7 total

| Day | Overnight | Miles | Notes |
| --- | --- | --- | --- |
| 77 | Miami | 26.2 | last 10.0 miles in Oklahoma |
| 78 | Miami | 26.1 | completed 2000 miles |

(first 7.9 miles in Oklahoma on Day 79)

*Chapter 6*

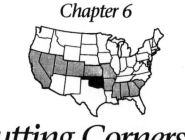

# Cutting Corners in Oklahoma

As if to perform a geographical balancing act, we immediately followed our longest-mileage state with our shortest. We would pay only a brief courtesy call on Oklahoma.

Between July 6 and July 8, we would clip the upper northeast corner of this state for a total of only 44 miles. But they'd be significant miles in that they'd push the total past 2000.

**DAY 77.** At 3:30 a.m. Elaine woke up and announced, "It's time to get the show on the road." My weary body objected, but I remembered we had a long way to drive to the start. The attraction today was that we'd exit Kansas and enter Oklahoma.

Given the early hour—a 4:40 start this time—and my need to warm up and shake out the kinks, the miles didn't add up very fast this morning. But they did come with considerably less stress to the body because of the lighter traffic and cooler weather.

Running along, I recalled a book I recently read by a guy who claimed to have run across the USA. Mile-wise, he did have sufficient distance to cross the country, but his route was not contiguous.

He would run some distance on a highway, then for various reasons he would leave the road, drive somewhere and run a number of miles on a high school track or in a parking lot or wherever he desired. Yet he insisted he ran across the USA and expressed resentment that anyone wouldn't accept his rationale.

By his standard, I could have escaped the biting flies in Kansas, the summits in Colorado and any distasteful roads in every state so far. Sorry, fella, but I can't buy your argument.

Can you believe Elaine and I are fantasizing about running from the Canadian to Mexican borders or the length of

California? One thing for sure, though: If we were to do either, about 20 miles a day would be my limit. We'd build in more play time!

Wildlife occupied my attention today, mainly because other attractions were lacking. Using my best Marine Corps scouting techniques, I quietly crossed a bridge and, looking up the creek, saw two big and healthy-looking deer.

I can't remember a day in the past two weeks when I've not heard the Bob White birds singing away all day. Could that same quartet have accompanied me for two weeks?

Before this trip, I'm not sure I even knew there was a Bob White bird. Now I'm always amused when I hear them sing, "Bob White" with a rising inflection on the "ite" syllable.

Man on a white horse, I came to the rescue of a turtle in mid-highway. I removed him to the safety of the nearby green grass.

With traffic light, I bravely—or maybe foolishly—ran on the right side of the road part of the day. I run better with my left leg up on the slope of the roadway.

I was blazing along at about a 12-minute-mile pace when a guy stopped to ask if I wanted a ride. Now, analyzing that, wouldn't I be in a hitchhiking posture rather than a running posture if I wanted a lift?

Minutes later, an elderly farmer brought his pickup to a screeching halt only inches away from me (my fault, since I was running with traffic), rattling me. Then he asked the inevitable, "Want a ride?" With two offers in such a short time, I must have looked weary.

In Chetopa, which bills itself as the "Catfish Capital" of the country, I made a phone call in another attempt to buy some shoes that fit. Two previous attempts had resulted in shoes being shipped to the wrong place.

This time, I talked with a supervisor who said, "We'll have the shoes sent to Cassville, Missouri. This will allow lead time for the shoes to arrive there before you do."

Now we face suspense until reaching Cassville four days from now. If the shoes arrive, dub this supervisor a miracle worker.

At the Oklahoma state line, Elaine and I took time out to camcord the border signs. We then passed farms all the way to Welch in the new state. On none of these farms did I see any of the heavy, expensive farm equipment prevalent in Kansas.

Approaching Welch, I followed a habit born of Kansas and looked for the water tower and grain elevator to signal the location of the town. Neither appeared. Another reminder that we weren't in Kansas anymore.

We're glad to be experiencing another state. Once we've cut across this corner of Oklahoma, the count will read six states down, six to go.

**DAY 78.** Last night, I did a quick and rough calculation. Today we would pass 2,000 miles, leaving about 1,200 yet to run.

At the rate of 26 miles a day, we are looking at 48 days to finish, which would be August 23. The trick is to keep the 26 miles going every day, to continue to resist the temptation to sleep in, and to take no days off. Hear me, will power?

It took all the will I could summon to be on the road at 4:40 a.m. today. For some reason, I was suffering from Delhi Belly at the start. It wasn't helped when I went by a hog farm. The odor was enough to wake a sleeping giant—or to get an old man to run faster in pursuit of fresh air.

Going by another hog farm, I observed the feeding system. There's food in an enclosed, circular bin that has a feeding trough around the bottom of it. Food is programmed to drop into different bins, making a thudding noise on arrival. Aware of this, the hogs stand around the trough and react with each thud. Hearing the noise, they run like hell to the feeder.

I eased past the first eight to 10 farmhouses today without a dog stirring. That would never have happened in Kansas.

Just as I was thinking that, out charged an Australian Shepherd. Well trained, he stopped at the property line. I had an experience with that breed of dog yesterday. The dog started charging towards me. I yelled to the farmer, "Is he friendly?" and the farmer nodded yes. Not bothering to brake, the dog jumped on me, wanting to be petted and wrestled. So we played fool-around.

Each time he bounced on me, I was knocked back a foot or two, and I marveled at his strength. A veritable Sherman tank, he was having a ball, and I was almost getting killed with affection.

The flies were after me today, seeking any blood the mosquitoes did not get. I went by an old horse in a pasture, and he was fighting flies. I could identify.

Passing one house, I watched four dogs so closely that I almost headed into an oncoming car. Near Miami (we're talking Oklahoma, not Florida), traffic was so thick that I made a career of jumping into the weeds.

These Okies (maybe I should be kinder and say "Sooners"!) are not about to move over for a runner. Come to think of it, I have yet to see another runner in this state.

As I waded through the weeds, I muttered at these primitive highway conditions. Could it be that too much of the Oklahoma tax money goes into the Sooner football program?

Today's drivers were the most inconsiderate and discourteous I've encountered in 2,000 miles. On one occasion, I was two feet out in the weeds and waiting for a semi to go by. The damn fool driver veered in my direction, crossing over the white fog line and onto the weeds, causing me to beat a hasty retreat.

I felt the hot draft of the truck as it pushed me a bit farther back and blew off my cap. "What the hell's wrong with this guy?" I wondered. Well, at least, I had cause to exercise some of my Marine Corps vocabulary.

The traffic conditions today were also stressful for Elaine. When we wrapped up the day, we decided that our best bet was to retreat to Miami and roost in the same spot as last night.

We wanted to get off the road as soon as possible. To this point, I rank Oklahoma on par with my Dehli Belly.

# E S S A Y

## The Spouse
by Elaine Reese

*(The bottom line in Elaine's role as contrasted with mine is that she did the drudgery, the yeoman work, while I was having the fun of playing kid, running, observing, meditating, and enjoying. The simple fact of the matter is that without her help, I would have faltered physically. Without her companionship, I would have been alone on an emotional roller-coaster without a partner to share the highs and lows. RUNXUSA mattered equally to each of us, and neither could let the other down. — Paul Reese.)*

Besides the twinkle in his eye, what first attracted me to Paul was the fact that he was so vitally alive. I soon discovered also that he is endowed with a spirit of adventure.

So I wasn't surprised when he proposed that we take a long, slow trip across the United States as soon as I retired. I had always planned to retire at 60, and I reached that golden age on March 10, 1990. I retired five days later, and our planning got underway—we would leave on our trip that April.

Two things I had always wanted when I retired were a small motor home, which I could drive, and a black Labrador puppy. We bought the motor home, but the dog would have to come later.

Paul would run his 25 to 26 miles each day. I would drive our new motor home and provide a full pit-crew service.

Since homemaking on the trip was to be my responsibility, I made the decision to keep the motor home as close as possible to a real home—rather than a camping-out home. This meant sheets and blankets, real dishes, pots and pans, and baking ingredients.

I'm a fanatic about baking my own cookies, coffee cake, etc. And since cleanliness is next to godliness, I was prepared for that, too. No small chore when a sweaty runner is hopping in and out of the motor home every hour the whole day long!

I took it upon myself to make home-cooked meals as much as possible and to have something yummy for Paul to eat at each of his pit stops. At first, I was showing off the variety of things I could prepare, even under rather primitive circumstances.

But after Paul tasted each one of my goodies, he added it to his mental menu and would ask for different types of tasty things at his pit stops. I became somewhat frustrated because there was no way I could have everything available for him at every pit stop—but I tried.

A part of the pit-crewing involved taking care of the motor home—checking the oil, water, and RV battery, washing outside windows, repairing screens that pulled loose, and so on. I located gasoline, propane, water, garbage cans, dump stations, mailboxes, grocery stores, telephones, laundromats and parking spots.

I also read maps and led Paul across the country. After a few mishaps, I learned to ask the natives if the road I was on was actually the road I THOUGHT I was on.

I lived in my little mobile cabin and moved it three miles down the road nearly every hour. While waiting for Paul to show up at the three-mile stops, I did a variety of things besides cleaning, cooking and servicing the motor home. I read books, I hand-sewed (no sewing machine) baby clothes for the soon-to-be grandchild, and a dress, a blouse and a purse for me. I crocheted, knitted, designed pig decorations and embroidered them on T-towels for home, and I practiced the guitar. I never did learn to play that thing!

I read my Bible every day, and played and sang hymns every Sunday. I wanted so much to take a day off, but I understood Paul's reasons for wanting to keep going everyday.

I listened to our battery radio, a gift from our children, and kept up on the news. I always had my eyes open for a *USA Today* newspaper because I knew Paul didn't want to lose touch with the world.

After George and Georgia Billingsley left us, I found myself very lonely without Georgia's company. I took up jogging each morning. It was really great to get out in the fresh air and see the trip from Paul's perspective. We had a chance to visit as we jogged along.

Since I was so alone on the trip, when I met any people I stopped for a short talk and told them all about RUNXUSA. This is one of the experiences I treasure most from the trip, meeting so many wonderful people.

Quite often, I had a cheering section lined up when Paul arrived for his pit stops. He always says, "You were my unauthorized PR crew."

# Overview of Missouri

**July 8 to July 14, 1990 — 169.3 miles — 2184.0 total**

| Day | Overnight | Miles | Notes |
| --- | --- | --- | --- |
| 79 | Neosho | 26.6 | last 18.7 miles in Missouri |
| 80 | near Cassville | 26.2 | took first wrong turn |
| 81 | Cape Fair | 26.6 | |
| 82 | Walnut Shade | 26.2 | |
| 83 | near Theodosia | 26.2 | |
| 84 | Bull Shoals Lk. | 26.2 | |

(first 19.2 miles in Missouri in Day 85)

*Chapter 7*

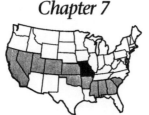

# *What Missouri Showed Me*

Passing into the lower Midwest would bring changes both positive and negative. On the plus side of the ledger: more towns to amble through and more farms to run past; more greenery to admire and more hour-by-hour changes in the scene.

The negatives: more cars on the roads in and around the towns and farms; more humidity in the air because of the wetter weather that spawns the greenery.

Missouri, where I'd run about 170 miles between July 8 and July 14, would be a homecoming of sorts for me. I had worked at the state's university in Columbia almost 30 years earlier.

**DAY 79.** One last thought about our short stay in Oklahoma: I went by many farmhouses, and dozens of dogs barked at me. But not one left the property line to pursue me. Oklahoma's dogs are well-trained and disciplined. I wish I could say the same for its drivers.

After yesterday's miserable running conditions, I busted my butt this early Sunday morning trying to get in some miles before the thundering herd hit the highways. The Missouri folk, I hope, will be more considerate than the Okies.

In 44 miles of Oklahoma, we didn't receive one offer of help or have anybody ask, "Do you have a problem?" Recall that in Kansas—in just one 26-mile day—I had had 13 such queries.

We didn't camcord at the Missouri border because there was no welcome-to sign. But this sign did appear: "Up to $1000 fine for littering and one year in jail."

Shortly after entering the new state, I passed a home with eight cars parked on the front lawn. Musta been a helluva party last night. No, no, not in Mizzou—probably a family reunion.

Coming back now to Missouri for the first time since 1961 conjures up memories of the three years I spent here. At that time, I was in the Marine Corps and was an associate professor at the University of Missouri, serving as executive officer of the Naval Reserve Officers Training Corps.

My boss was Captain Albert Pelling, USN, a remarkable and likeable gentleman. My warm memories revolve around experiences with the midshipmen, particularly those who played for our Navy basketball team which won the NROTC championship (17 schools), and which played college freshmen teams.

I still keep in touch with one of the midshipmen, Ray Vickery, who owns a newspaper in Salem, Missouri. He had hoped to visit Elaine and me on this trip but couldn't make it because the Missouri Newspaper Publishers Association (of which he was president) was holding a convention.

The others were: George Peters, a stock broker in St. Louis; Jerry Everman, an engineer with General Electric; twins John and Gerald McGee, engineers whose initial job interviews were with Admiral Rickover (they got the job); Joe Yeager, an airline pilot, and Ron Stout, a turkey farmer in Missouri.

My early running in Missouri today was as pleasant as my memories of this state. Highway 10 couldn't have been much better—a breakdown lane to myself, the road flat, the traffic light.

Were the conditions like this all the way to Charleston, I could pick up a couple of days. The stress factor here was zero.

Running along this morning, facing the sun, I thought that an appropriate title for a west-to-east transcon run might be, *Sun in My Face.* But *Left Leg Down* might be more suited to running and, besides, it sounds suspiciously sexy.

I found myself wondering why my equilibrium is so much better when I am on the right side of the road running with traffic than when I am on the left side facing traffic. Does it have anything to do with which leg is up and which is down?

The highway was so deserted that I could stop for a bladder matter without taking camouflage. No way would I go out into the weeds since Charlie Mersereau, a Missouri friend, had warned me that the Missouri weeds are filled with chiggers.

The early-morning reverie over the great road conditions didn't last out the day. On Highway 60, I suddenly encountered 15 cars approaching me bumper to bumper at 70 miles per hour.

Then, unbelievably, one crazy driver among them swerved into the breakdown lane, passing all the others on the right and heading directly for me. Luckily, I had time to hop into the weeds (chiggers be damned!).

The lesson here: always run against traffic. Had this scenario developed when I was running with traffic, I would not have seen that klunkhead in the breakdown lane and, most likely, he would have spotted me just about the time he hit me.

My right knee flickered a few times today. I tried to do a heap of disassociating—wondering how I'd spend the $10 million won in the California lotto—and this helped make the miles easier. If a runner associates only—dwells on miles and his injuries—that will tire him.

I find it's usually around the 11-mile mark that I get a bit discouraged. The thinking is: "I've run my butt off, only got 11 miles done and have a heaping 15 to do." However, once at 15 miles, I pick up on positive thinking.

A positive thought to end the day: Again this morning when I woke up, I had stomach cramps. But unlike yesterday, when I began running, they disappeared. This might sound silly, but I suspect that the way my metabolism is working, I need food in the middle of the night.

**DAY 80.** For the first time in three days, I started without a stomach cramp. Maybe that banana I ate in the middle of the night helped.

By now, you've guessed that the nearest thing to heaven for us is a back country road—the less traveled the better. Late yesterday and again today, it took the form of Road D.

Out here, with the world still asleep and me awake and active, I own this territory. Of course, the birds were out and chirping—including a Bob White with a lisp. I went by a chicken ranch where the roosters were competing to see which could be the top cockle-doodle-do.

One difference between the rural areas in Missouri and Kansas is that now there are 10 houses for every one we saw in Kansas over the same distance. But there seemed to be more affluence among the Kansas farmers.

I've not yet seen any high-powered farm equipment on these Missouri farms like that in Kansas. There seems to be a farmhouse about every half-mile, so the land holdings can't be very big. And for every farm, a dog.

I passed a turkey farm and saw a thousand or more white birds in a huge poultry shed, 100 or so yards long. They stood bumper to bumper, gobbling and staring out from the enclosure.

A farm or two later, the same thing, but this time the shed's inhabitants were white chickens. A sign advertised a poultry shed for sale and claimed it holds 12,500 birds.

In the running world in which I dwell, there are good days and bad days. Today, both knees gave me trouble. Once, a feeling like an electric shock went through my left knee, buckling it. I momentarily stumbled but didn't fall. After walking a few steps, I resumed running without a problem. Wish I understood what's going on with that knee.

I do marvel somewhat at how both knees have held up so long. I'm praying they'll stay afloat for 1,200 or so miles to the finish of this clambake.

For one of the few times in 2,000 miles covered, I missed a turn today. I'd gone three-fourths of a mile out of the way before realizing my mistake. Beating a hasty retreat, I bemoaned the wasted time and energy.

But at least I kept moving. It was somewhat sad today to see so many homes with older people—60 and upwards—sitting in a chair on the front porch or in a yard and watching the world go by. This is their day. Seems a waste of body and brain.

I got a kick out of the looks the older Missouri farmers in their pickups gave me. They seemed to say, "What in the hell are you doing running out here in this heat, old man?"

While Elaine was parked for a pit stop, a lady came out to talk with her about our motor home and they chatted about our run. The lady took off for Wheaton to tell the local press.

Half an hour later, the newspaper folks caught up with Elaine and interviewed her. Then they tracked me down for a photo. We've never sought publicity but don't mind admitting that we enjoy these rare and brief moments of fame.

I'm left with a good feeling today because I managed to run at least 85 percent of the distance despite a couple of complaining knees. Then we drove into Cassville for Christmas in July.

After three failed attempts, the mail finally brought a new pair of New Balance 840 shoes that FIT. Sayonara, cut-out toes!

**DAY 81.** I spent a lot of energy today moving from side to side on the road to avoid cars and to stay out of the chigger-loaded weeds. On reflection, maybe I was unkind to Kansas in criticizing its narrow roads. Missouri's state highways seem the same: narrow, no paved shoulder or bike lane.

I learned the hard way during this zigzagging that Missouri has unmarked police cars. This discovery unfolded as I approached a black pickup parked beside the road. The driver beckoned to me like a teacher motioning to an elementary student. I asked, "Do you want to talk with me?" He nodded yes. "I have a complaint about you jumping in front of a gravel truck," he announced.

Seeing the radar on his dashboard, I asked if he was a police officer and got a confirmation. I was irked—first, because of his uncouth approach (fingering to me as if I were a child); second, because the report was stupid (I crossed the road safely, to escape the gravel that the truck was spewing); third, because this guy was acting like Mr. Superior.

But I played his game, even listening to him telling me this was not a good road to "jog" on. Finally, he dismissed me by saying, "You may leave now."

Though sizzling, I had managed to keep my cool. Lucky I had, because if I'd given this guy any back talk, he probably would have taken pleasure in jailing me.

I suspect he was from the local sheriff's department and not the Missouri Highway Patrol. The Patrol has more class than that.

This incident aside, today's rural mountain setting was truly enjoyable to run. We're into the Ozarks now.

Elaine was taken with the scenery, too. But her joy was tempered by the stress of driving the curvy mountain roads. This was one of those days when she was happier than I to see our workday end.

**DAY 82.** A couple of miles out of Cape Fair, near Table Rock Lake, we were again on a curvy, narrow road enclosed by forests on both sides. Beautiful, but dangerous and difficult running.

Missouri must have a vehicle code like that of Kansas: if you can afford a yellow light atop your vehicle, you are entitled to use it.

All day, the Missouri farmhouses continued to be no more than half a mile apart. The range in home quality was widespread. Some were luxurious ($200,000 to $300,000, expensive in these parts), some squalid, and the rest middle-class abodes.

Going into Reed Springs, I found myself on a flat road with a straight stretch for a half-mile. Unbelievable after all the hills. A resort town, Reed Springs, gave the impression of being an overgrown concession stand. Obviously, it exists for the tourist trade, and the stores and shops reflect that.

By far the most impressive sight was a luxury home in the middle of town. One of its distinctive features was its high metal fences, designed so that a team of German Shepherd dogs—I saw four of them on duty—could patrol it. (A local citizen told me that the four doghouses I saw have heating and air conditioning, and hot and cold water.)

A second feature was a huge waterfall design with an enormous eagle ornament sitting atop it. Also evident were surveillance cameras. All of which made me wonder: what retired Mafia man lives here?

With the hustle of traffic, getting through town was a pain in the ass. We wanted to camcord the Mafia house, but parking was impossible.

I was daydreaming while leaving town and started to go west on Highway 160. Elaine, waiting at the road junction to check on me, honked to get me turned around and headed in the right direction.

This was one of those days when I forced myself from one pit stop to the next. All the traffic dampened my sense of humor. But I did manage to smile at a sign that read, "Don't drive like hell through God's country."

This has been sort of an oddball day. Overcast all day and muggy, the sun never coming out. Depressing weather.

The two towns we went through—Cape Fair and Reed Springs—were not special except for the Mafia house. We were in greenery and forest growth most of the day, but it was not as striking as yesterday.

It's been a day without much memorable. But I wound up happy since I was still able to run through some distress signals from latent injuries.

**DAY 83.** This morning, I lacked the energy and desire to cross back and forth on the road to avoid cars. So I held my own on the road, claiming a small piece of real estate and forcing the cars to move over in sort of a Russian roulette maneuver.

In two hours of playing this game, I waved to every driver who moved over. With the exception of one senior citizen, all returned the wave.

I disassociated from running by thinking about our finish. At this stage of our endeavor, Elaine and I have definitely decided not to end at Savannah.

We're now considering three alternate sites, all in South Carolina: Marine Corps Air Station at Beaufort, Marine Corps Recruit Depot at Parris Island and Hilton Head Island.

I dodged traffic again through the resort town of Forsyth,

on Shadow Rock Lake. The town was entirely without personality—simply a shopping center along the highway, bedecked with an inordinate number of motels. Despite the traffic problem, though, it is always nice to go through a small town, get a feel for the community, and inject some diversity into the running day.

East of Forsyth, I saw the aftermath of recent flooding. Many buildings in the lake recreational area had water to their rooftops. On a basketball court, water stood at hoop level.

At a scenic overlook, Elaine talked to some people from Illinois, telling them about our run. They responded by telling her about their 82-year-old father in Illinois, who works a wheat farm all by himself and adamantly refuses to install air conditioning in his combine. Hey, in nine years I could be operating a wheat farm!

Going along later, I felt something licking my ankle. "Can't be, must be hallucinating," I thought.

Then I looked down, and here was this little Welsh Terrier trotting along and licking away. He was a classy little gentleman.

I petted him, gave him some attention, and told him, "Now go home." But as I took off, he followed.

Afraid a car would hit him because he was so small and hard to see, I picked him up, carried him back across the road to his house, and deposited him with the command, "Stay!"

This pooch had a mind of his own. He again followed me.

"Okay," I thought, "I'll run away from the little sucker." I ran my butt off for half a mile, only to find him still on my heels.

Luckily, I came upon Elaine, waiting at a pit stop. I told her, "Meet Mr. McGillicuddy. The guy loves me. I can't shake him."

I entered the motor home for the pit stop and noticed Mr. McGillicuddy waiting patiently outside. Elaine and I discussed tactics to escape him and came up with a plan.

Elaine would take a piece of meatloaf to the rear of the motor home and entertain our new friend while I sneaked out the front and down the highway. The plan worked, except that in the process of going through the grass to the highway I encountered a big black snake (three feet of snake is huge to me), jumped, and came close to tripping in the weeds. Once on the highway, I was airborne.

Elaine left Mr. McGillicuddy to savor the meatloaf. I prayed that the elegant little gentleman made it home safely up the highway. He was a delightful companion who obviously enjoyed our company—and the treat he'd worked so hard to earn.

Late in the day, an Ozark man in a sputtering pickup was kind enough to stop and ask, "Do you need a ride, or are you just out jogging?" Let's don't make this complicated, I thought before replying, "Just out jogging."

"Okay," he said, driving away. Now I wish I had his name and address so I could buy him a new pickup when I win $10 or $20 million in the California lotto.

As I go through Missouri, the opinion I formed of the rural folks during the three years I lived here is reinforced. They are sturdy people, they can weather a storm, their basic values are good, and they are people of character.

All told, this has been a pleasant day, varied somewhat with the mountains, the flood scenes, the resort towns and the mild weather. It's satisfying for me that I was able to run every segment even though my energy reservoir seemed to be drained.

The trick is to hang on like this for 41 more days. By now, I've learned that the secret is to take them one day at a time.

**DAY 84.** A little excitement during the drive to the start this morning. First, Elaine had to slam on her brakes to avoid hitting a skunk on the road.

He then got under the motor home, soon came out in front of it, and led us down the highway for 50 yards. He was primed for firing but, thankfully, never unloaded.

Random thoughts from today's early miles:

* Once again, I take my hat off to UPS. I went by an open ranch gate and saw a sign reading "UPS pickup." I looked down the road, out into the hills, and it was almost a mile to the house. How can UPS make money on that deal?

* I can vouch for one thing about the people in this part of the state: They like ornamental deer. I swear that along Highway 160 I've seen about a hundred homes with them on their front lawn.

* I'm beginning to think that pigs must be romantically inclined. This occurred to me as I went by a pen and saw two different couples embracing.

* As I go along, there's not time for everything I'd like to do, like stopping to pet the horse I saw this morning. Evidently lonesome, it moved along the fence line to follow me.

My mental meanderings were interrupted when a Chevrolet at least a decade old screeched to a halt. Its woman driver smiled, revealing some missing teeth, and announced, "Your wife is on her way out to meet you. She's about a mile away."

I thanked her for the information. Elaine soon appeared,

taking her morning jog with a dog in tow.

He was a mutt of many varieties, so I named him "Heinz." He responded by jumping all over me and demanding attention. He then followed us back to the motor home 1-1/2 miles away.

After my pit stop, Heinz was still there. So we repeated the trick used yesterday on Mr. McGillicuddy.

I give Heinz half a chicken sandwich. Gulp and gone! Probably a mistake, because then he took off with me.

I repeatedly commanded, "Stay!" and "Go home!" His response was to turn mournful eyes to me as if to say, "I thought you were my friend."

I surrendered, and he followed me for more than a half-hour until we came to a country store. Something distracted him there, and I lost him.

Elaine said, "I saw his master leave for work, so my guess is that he chose us as his entertainment for the day." One thing for sure, I didn't have to worry about this guy getting home safely. He's street-wise.

Another thing for sure: he's better equipped to do 26 miles than I.

Later, I did my good deed for the day. I spotted, by actual count, 14 cans of beer that had never been opened. So I stopped an Ozark gent in a pickup and told him about this treasure. Minutes later, I saw him picking up the beer.

A bit of a scare after the last pit stop. Elaine had no sooner driven away when I realized that I could barely walk on my left foot. Felt like a damaged bone, but it was probably arthritis.

My first remedial action was to lace the shoestring tighter. I walked gingerly and then gradually eased into a jog on the uphill, which seemed to help. In 10 minutes, I had it back to normal and resumed running. I suspect this trouble resulted from my inactivity during the pit stop.

Near the end of today's trek, I crossed a long bridge over Bull Shoals Lake. A humorous thought crossed my mind: a transcon run could be enlivened with the requirement that the runner swim all bodies of water encountered.

Crossing the country my way is taxing enough, thank you. Somebody I talked with recently asked, "Do you ever think about quitting?"

I simply replied, "Not yet, at least." Truth of the matter is, the only stopper would be if I could not move forward. That includes moving on crutches if necessary.

Around the time we had logged the first 1,000 miles, I

asked Elaine, "What would you do if I said I was going to quit?" She replied, "You mean because you were ill or injured?"

"No, " I said, "just tired of running." She said, "I'd kick your butt out the door and tell you to get running." Hey, that's my kind of girl!

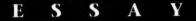

# E  S  S  A  Y

## *The Patient*

by Frank J. Boutin, M.D., and Robert D. Boutin, M.D.

*(Frank Boutin is an orthopedic surgeon who has treated my injuries—both running and non-running—for more than 20 years. His son, Robert Boutin, is a diagnostic radiologist and avid triathlete. — Paul Reese.)*

Running across the United States is a rare accomplishment at any age. At 73, this feat is nothing less than phenomenal—especially considering the fact that the average lifespan for men in the very country Paul Reese ran across is 72.3 years.

Exercise, however, is not a miracle drug. Despite its numerous beneficial effects, it is not without potential hazards. Paul is a striking example of how running can produce long-lasting health benefits and enriching personal experiences, but can also be the cause of frustrating injuries.

Most of Paul's orthopedic problems during his 30-year running career have been related to the repetitive stresses that a long-distance runner of any age places on his muscles, tendons, ligaments and bones. The type of overuse injuries that he experienced illustrate the types of setbacks an ambitious athlete may suffer.

Feet take a great pounding and must be protected with good footwear. Plantar fasciitis bothered Paul after a marathon in 1979. It responded to use of an orthotic with a varus wedge.

At times after races in 1981-82, Paul experienced a variety of pains in his feet. These especially bothered him after his 100-mile run over mountains and valleys from Squaw Valley to Auburn, California, in June 1981. He accommodated by using a soft Spenco orthotic and lacing the running shoes tightly, as the hard orthotics cut his heels on the irregular terrain.

The knee is one of the most commonly injured areas in runners. One of the knee injuries which Paul has sustained is called "iliotibial band friction syndrome." The iliotibial band is a large ligament connecting the ilium (part of the pelvis) with the tibia (one of the shin bones). Fortunately, only once has this condition disabled him enough to require modification of his training.

Other types of knee injuries have also affected Paul. He was temporarily slowed by patello-femoral irritation (between the kneecap and the end of the thigh bone) after racing a hilly 50 miles in 1985. Paul responded well to appropriate exercises and the avoidance of bent-knee activities for several days.

Injuries to his medial menisci (at the inner aspect of his knee joints) occurred in 1973 and again in 1989. Each injury forced a modification of Paul's running for two to three months.

Paul has suffered hip pain caused by trochanteric bursitis, an inflammation of the soft-tissue pad which lies between the iliotibial band and the upper-outer aspect of the thigh bone. This overuse injury slowed his activity for a short time in 1973 and again in 1980, but ultimately resolved.

The lower-back pain that Paul periodically experiences while running is caused by a condition called "spondylolysis." This refers to a stress fracture in the arch of one of the vertebral bones which makes up the spine. With each heel strike while running, the unstable spine segment is jarred, potentially resulting in pain.

When Paul experiences low-back pain from this condition, his discomfort can be ameliorated by a sacroiliac belt, which provides local stability to the spine without interfering with his running. Aside from this pathological area at the lower end of the spine, the remaining levels on X-ray suggest the spine of a young man.

One of Paul's more acute and debilitating injuries occurred during a race in 1988. All of a sudden, without warning, in the first half-mile of an 8-K race, he felt a tremendous tearing sensation deep in the lower part of his buttock. Paul fell to the ground involuntarily and could not finish the race.

Subsequent physical examination and magnetic resonance imaging (MRI) showed that he had torn the left hamstring tendons near their origin on the ischial tuberosity (sit-down bone). Trying to return to running six weeks later, he could still only shuffle 100 yards, but he gradually returned to normal racing over the next two months.

Runners are determined people, as exemplified by Paul's having been struck by a car while running a race in 1968. He was thrown an estimated 40 feet but was able to get up and finish the race.

In 1974, Paul fell while running and struck his right chest against a rock. He sustained multiple rib fractures and pneumothorax (air in the pleural space between the chest wall and the lung, due to the sharp spikes of ribs puncturing the lung). He finished his run before being taken to the hospital for insertion of a lung suction tube to remove the air and expand the lung.

He did miss the Dipsea Run over Mount Tamalpais in 1979 due to fractured ribs resulting from a white-water river run. Multiple rib fractures a few days before the 1980 Boston Marathon slowed his time to 3:19 in that race, but did not keep him from running and finishing.

Paul has never allowed a few aches and pains, or his asthma, to interfere with his daily runs. His philosophy is that we will be much happier and healthier as we grow older if we participate in aerobic sports rather than sitting in a rocking chair watching the world go by us during our limited remaining days.

# *Overview of Arkansas*

**July 14 to July 23, 1990 — 238.9 miles — 2422.9 total**

| Day | Overnight | Miles | Notes |
|-----|-----------|-------|-------|
| 85 | Lakeview | 26.2 | last 7.0 miles in Arkansas |
| 86 | Norfolk Dam | 26.3 | temperature hit 103 degrees |
| 87 | Melbourne | 26.5 | |
| 88 | Batesville | 26.2 | |
| 89 | near Newport | 26.1 | |
| 90 | near McCory | 26.2 | |
| 91 | near Brinkley | 26.3 | |
| 92 | Clarendon | 26.6 | RUNXUSA three months old |
| 93 | Helena | 26.3 | |

(first 21.4 miles in Arkansas on Day 94)

*Chapter 8*

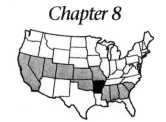

# *Arkansas Traveling*

Into the South! Here we would stay until this journey ended in about a month.

But one month of running still would require about 800 miles on the road. Anything could still happen in those hot, humid, hilly, heavily trafficked miles.

Arkansas would reduce that mileage-to-go by nearly 240 between July 14 and July 23. But I couldn't afford to be dwelling too much on the finish line still several states away.

**DAY 85.** A lively beginning to our day. When we came out at 4:30 a.m. to unhook our motor home, five skunks were gathered by our rear tires. We were within two or three feet of them before our flashlights revealed their presence.

Elaine yelled, "Get out of here, little skunkies. Go on. Get back in your hole. Shoo, shoo!" Magic words because, tails arched, they all retreated into a culvert.

Another hilly start, which made for a punishing warmup. Same narrow road with no shoulder. I was bordering the grass and weeds, not in them, but I swear I could feel those damn chiggers chomping on my ankles.

By mid-morning, we'd gone from light to moderate to heavy traffic. Everybody was in a helluva hurry, including the guy hauling his pigs to the bacon-makers and the guy towing his boat in a frenzy to get it into the water.

By now, I've come to expect Saturday—with all its frantic recreational travel—to be more stressful than the other days. And this was a Saturday like all the others.

As I approached the Arkansas state line, I noticed four pubs all bunched together on the Missouri side, along with a couple of places selling lottery tickets. There must have been a message here about liquor and lottery sales in Arkansas.

Elaine and I stopped at the border for our usual stateline camcording. Going into Arkansas, my thoughts centered on the basics: "Nine-and-a-half days to clear the state if we're lucky. Wonder how the roads will be. How many Highway Patrol officers will we encounter, and will they give us any grief?"

Let's hear it for Arkansas. The first road in the new state was blacktop, newly surfaced, and it had a one-foot paved shoulder. Sheer luxury!

The biggest Arkansas surprise today was the quality of its roads—better than either Kansas or Missouri. But for some reason, I wasn't excited about coming into Arkansas—at least to the same degree that I had been on arrival in other states.

Could be that I'm somewhat concerned over the problem I've had the past couple of days. Something is out of whack, because I've urinated at least 20 times a day.

The question is why: (1) bad water; (2) not sweating since the past two days have been cold; (3) bladder infection; (4) some fallout from my prostatic cancer and radiation; (5) reaction to some non-alcoholic beer we've been drinking?

Elaine swung over to Mountain Home to collect our mail before the post office closed early on this Saturday. Some of the mail we'd expected wasn't there. Following normal procedure, she left a forwarding address down the road a piece.

The best way to sum up this day, as I write in an RV park beside the White River, is by saying that I am glad to have it behind me.

**DAY 86.** Seems I'm due again for stream-of-consciousness writing. Reporting an occasional day this way gives the most accurate picture of what I do, see, and think out here on the road.

Starting this morning near Mountain Home, I'm impressed with all the forestation in this area. It's a far cry from the scenic mountains of the West but easier on the weary old body. It's cold enough—at least for a gent of three score and 13—for a polypro top and a light windbreaker suit.

I'm going by the most attractive site yet in Mountain Home. It turns out to be the Baxter Memorial Cemetery, which has a building on it that resembles Mount Vernon and is identified as the Roller Funeral Home.

I gotta get moving. My tired body might be tempted to go no farther, settling into eternal rest here. But, Lord, I'm not ready! Are we ever?

This is unbelievable—I go by a furniture store at 7:07 a.m. As expected, it's closed, but 20 or more new outdoor furniture pieces sit on the sidewalk out front.

I see no security evident. What do we have here, honest citizens or an efficient police force?

Exiting Mountain Home on Highway 5 south, I pass the South Side Baptist Church. In a town like this, there are also North Side, East Side and West Side Baptist churches.

I'm conscious of something different about this morning's traffic. Then I realize that, unlike yesterday, few cars are towing boats.

Today, we have many drivers in their Sunday duds heading for town. Since most are senior citizens, a good guess is that they're church-goers.

I come out from my second pit stop, start to run and am whammied with stomach cramps. Could it be because I'm running too soon after gulping down some lasagna?

Odd observation: It seems that 25 percent of the litter I see comes from McDonald's. Is that a barometer of the clientele? And the odd part is that there are not that many McDonald's along our route.

Finally, stomach cramps gone and bladder problems abated (oh, the ravages of age!), I'm back into some steady running. Oh, la, la! Feels good!

The thought crosses my mind that running across the USA is a pass-or-fail course. You make it, or you don't. There's always the anxiety that some latent injury will pop out to stop you.

At Salesville, we depart Highway 5 (oh, I'll miss that paved shoulder!) and take Highway 177 (which doesn't even show on the AAA maps) to experience the adventure of another back road. A sign tells me that Norfork Dam is two miles away. Translation: watch out for recreational traffic.

As I approach the dam, I see a Corps of Engineers campground at its base. Could be our home for the night.

At the base of Norfork Dam, where the road divides, I stop an Arkansas driver and ask, "Which one of these roads goes to Jordan?" He growls an answer. What a contrast, I'm thinking, to the fine folks of Nevada, Utah, Kansas and Missouri.

As I cross the roadway over the dam, it's surprising to look at the huge lake and to see only four boats on it. In California, there would be dozens.

It's pleasant crossing the dam since I can run in a four-foot breakdown lane. I'll have to remember to compliment Elaine on plotting this scenic route. The run through this area has added meaning to the day.

I run on another 10 miles. With no other prospects on the horizon, Elaine and I decide to drive back to the Corps of Engineers campground at Norfork Dam to spend the night in a pleasant setting that the AAA maps and the Good Sam campground book neglect to mention.

**DAY 87.** What a delightful feeling it was to step out of the motor home early this morning and to start running without any injury alerts. No nagging warning, "Hey, watch out for me, treat me tenderly."

For a long time, I've harbored the urge to take a day off and rest. But I don't for three reasons:

1. It would skew the physiological test of what a 73-year-old can or can't do.

2. It would take some of the challenge out of the enterprise.

3. If I did skip a day, I might have a helluva time restarting. Rest could be habit-forming.

This keep-going attitude is as tough on Elaine as it is on me. I give her a lot of credit for going along with my wish not to call timeout.

This leads again to the thought that there are two approaches to running across the USA. One is to be obsessed with speed and miles. The other is to go along at a more leisurely pace, and to appreciate all the sights and scenery rather than making time and mileage the prime focus. Even while insisting on running every day, I favor the slow-down-and-see approach.

I must mention that in the last 75 miles I've seen at least 25 antique stores. We're talking quantity here, not quality.

The town of Pineville that I passed through early today was unusual in that, with a population of 193, it had a pawn shop. And sitting on the front yard of a home was a 1962 red Impala in mint condition and for sale. In California, it would be gobbled up.

Near Calico Rock, I went by a beautiful brick mansion set amidst a grove of pine trees. The acreage alone in California would cost a quarter-million or more.

By contrast, a short while later I saw a place that was straight out of the movie, "Deliverance." Four shacks on this property; junk strewn in all directions; windows covered with blankets, paper, foil, anything but curtains, and four beat-up cars in various stages of disintegration.

On down the road a piece, atop a hill, sat another lovely brick home. Welcome to Arkansas!

Nary a day goes by, it seems, without a report of a near-miss on the highway. Today was no exception.

I heard a truck coming up the hill as I was going with traffic, so I crossed to the left side and a bit off the road before the truck went by. Just as it passed me, I turned to look back and was aghast to see a woman driver heading straight toward me. Instantly, I jumped another two feet out into the weeds and unleashed a litany of locker-room language.

Obviously, she had been following the truck so closely that she didn't see me until she was upon me while making her illegal pass over a double line. The happy sequel to this story was that, a few miles down the road, Elaine saw an Arkansas Highway Patrolman issuing this woman a ticket.

Let me tell you, when a guy sees a car descending on him at 65 miles an hour, he pumps a heap of adrenaline. If I want to survive this highway-running venture, I'd better realize that if something stupid can be done by a driver, it will be.

After thinking that, I witnessed a tragedy in the making. A man drove by me in a pickup with four little kids in the back, all six and younger, a couple of them sitting on the ledge of the truck bed. It seemed inevitable that one of them would tumble out onto the highway.

A first for us today: Elaine stopped to buy propane near the town of Melbourne. When she told the owner about our run, he refused payment. After finishing, we returned to Melbourne and went to City Hall (which consisted of one room with two desks) and asked about RV hookups. We learned that only parking and water were available, but accepted the invitation to make ourselves at home under the water tower in the city park.

**DAY 88.** Overnight, Elaine and I were introduced to the Arkansas cousin of the cricket. This unidentified critter—well, more precisely, a whole team of them—conversed noisily throughout the night. Elaine thought they sounded like a dozen angry rattlesnakes. Their symphony was unlike anything we'd ever heard before.

I've learned not to prejudge the day by how I feel at its start. Running in darkness at the start, I had a hard time shaking out the kinks. But once all body components awakened, I ran without difficulty.

I ran about 85 percent of the route today with no body part clamoring for attention.

My daily pit stops have two constants: Elaine always has some tasty treat, and when I emerge from the motor home and hit the road I must ease back into running. My overworked old body solidifies quickly.

It was obvious from the start today that traffic would be a problem. We traveled a commute road to Batesville, which, with a population of 8000-plus, is big in this part of the country.

Once again, this was a narrow, curvy, hilly road. Many of the homes along this route flew the Arkansas state flag, a cousin of the Confederate banner.

The gravel truck shuttle accompanied us again. Every time a truck approached, I jumped into the weeds a couple of feet because I knew the driver would make no effort to move over or to reduce speed. Fact is, instead of moving away from me, these drivers tended to inch closer to the outer edge of the road so I'd have to leap farther onto the shoulder. Since this happened so regularly, I decided they'd pegged me as their day's entertainment.

General comment on drivers: From the experience of 2270 miles on the road, I'd rate young men as the most alert drivers... young women as driving beyond their capabilities, often misjudging speed and curving... old ladies as dangerous because of their poor reaction time, judgment of distance and tendency to panic. As for old men, their driving abilities span so wide a range—from the downright dangerous to being on a par with young men—that they can't be categorized.

Ten miles into today's run, I came upon a construction zone where I spent the better part of an hour. The new road was blacktop with lanes wider than usual. One fringe benefit of these zones is that I often run unmolested because cars are prohibited.

Passing through Springmill, I detoured from the road to read that the town was founded in 1867 by a Confederate colonel. The mill is still in service, the last of its type operating in Arkansas.

Down the road a bit, I noticed a small creek, about three feet wide, flowing between the edge of the forestation and the bottom of the highway drop. The water was crystal clear. Had the temperature been only a bit warmer, I would have become a biathlete and made the transition from running to swimming.

As it was, I held off becoming a swimmer until we reached the pool at our destination—an RV park in Batesville.

**DAY 89.** Surprised, as I started at 5:20 this morning, to find a muscle pull in my right groin. That pain gradually eased, but I wasn't out of the woods yet because then my left foot started giving me fits.

If it's not one thing, it's another. Just as the foot pain waned, a muscle in my upper left leg hampered me for a few miles. Strangely, it felt better when I ran than when I walked, so I ran through it.

Most of today, I plodded along like a robot. Nothing wrong with that as long as there's no mechanical failure.

It's blessings-counting time: Today's road conditions for running were the best that I can remember for a long time— less hilly, less curvy. Maybe the flat road allowed me to run through the groin, foot, and quad problems. I wonder.

Memorable sights from another day on the road:

* The long uphill climb out of Batesville which rewarded me with a splendid view of the town and the White River valley.

* Elaine's first pit stop by a cemetery. Every time she makes such a stop, I pray that it has no symbolic meaning.

* Down the road a piece (as they say in Arkansas), two impressive sights in Rosie (Where do they get the names for these hamlets? Another was called "Oil Trough!"): a home with an excellent tennis court and another with a large pool. This in a town with a total of five houses.

* Ponds on many of the ranches. Ponds 30 or 40 yards across, at which I saw cows cooling and people fishing.

* A crop-duster doing his thing in a stubby biplane. He made his run, dusting, with his wheels barely above the ground, then pulled up and banked sharply left, pulled up to desired altitude, then turned right and came around for another run. Very efficient use of air space.

* Another first: the sign read "Quail Farm," and I saw that it sold dressed birds, eggs and baby quail.

* Running by 30 or so dogs without incident. One pack of six had me concerned enough to stop and pick up a stick, but they soon scrambled off in hot pursuit of a dog in heat.

* Finishing near Newport, a hodge-podge town where zoning seems non-existent. The downtown business section is minimal. The shopping action is on the outskirts of town.

I ran tired today but on the philosophy, "You gotta believe." If you believe in it, you can do it. It's down there in the well, waiting for me to draw it out.

**DAY 90.** My thoughts go back to Jacksonport State Park where we spent last night. In addition to us, there were only two other parties camped at this beautiful spot on the White River.

Again I find myself comparing this park with those in California, where you'd need to reserve a spot three weeks in advance and pay $10 just to pitch a tent. In Arkansas, the charge for an electric and water hookup is $5.

Near Newport early this morning, I felt a bit shaky because I'd already seen the two bridges to be crossed. Both had only two lanes and about six inches of space between the road's edge and the bridge rail.

The first bridge was about a quarter-mile long and the second a half-mile. My only course of action, if I encountered an oncoming car, would have been to jump to the rail and hug it. But I must be leading a charmed life, because I only met two cars on these bridges and both drivers gave me a wide berth. Nonetheless, I felt relief at putting these obstacles behind me.

Two strange sights seen in Newport while the town still slept. First, I stopped to study a fire in the downtown section. A building had been demolished, and whatever was combustible had been subsequently burned on the spot. Can't get away with that in many places nowadays. Later, I saw a chicken scampering about. Don't see that in many downtown areas.

Today's driver-watching observations: I'm beginning to notice that 80 percent of the men driving pickups in Arkansas have beards. Make of that what you will.

As I go along, I'm pleased to note how many of the black drivers wave to me. I've seen about 10 times as many black people in Arkansas as in any state since we left California.

I stopped to talk with a farmer who was spraying his soybeans. His machine intrigued me. The front part looked like a small airplane cockpit. Behind it, at right angle to the fuselage, was a long metal pipe, and from the pipe came a number of faucets dispensing the spray. "We call this contraption a 'Spray Coupe'," he told me.

Wish I could figure out what triggers my energy level. In no particular pattern, it goes up and down, down and up at different times during each day and from day to day.

On my mind now is the map work that I want to do tonight. I'm anxious to compute how many miles we have left to the Atlantic and then translate that to days of running, because I feel that my luck with good health can't last forever. So far, I've been blessed.

**DAY 91.** I did a quick calculation last night and figured that, including today, we have 867 miles to go. This translates to 33 days at the rate of 26 miles a day. Hopefully, that is the max.

Strange how, prior to this trek, contemplating 867 miles of running would have been almost frightening. Now it simply reduces to 33 days on the road, which—barring injury or getting splattered by a car—feels well within my reach.

At today's start, I wondered how drained Elaine and I would feel from last night's experience. Without a hookup in 90-degree-plus weather, the motor home stayed sweating hot until about 11 p.m.

However, we did have some good entertainment. First, a crop-duster performed in the field across the road until darkness fell, making a couple of passes that almost clipped the trees under which we sat.

Once it got dark, the lightning bugs doing their aerobatics at tree height fascinated Elaine, who stayed up late watching their antics. Finally, the Arkansas cousins to the cricket kept up their chorus all evening.

Elaine must be getting desperate for companionship. She asked today, "Can you look for a small turtle for me?"

Too bad she didn't tell me that a week or two ago when turtles were plentiful along the road. Now, finding a live turtle will be a good trick, since we've seen only one in the last 100 miles. Nonetheless, I've gone on turtle patrol.

This wouldn't be the time for Elaine to renew her campaign for a puppy. I wasn't too kindly disposed to dogs today. Just as I was thinking, "Hey, I've gone 11 miles without any trouble from a dog," one with a nasty disposition charged out at me. A lady at the house yelled, "Pappy!" but he paid no attention to her.

He got within six feet of me before obeying my menacing, "Stay!" The lady called again, he retreated, and she spanked him while saying, "Bad dog"—all for my benefit, I assume.

A sociological note: Seventy percent of the cars I saw this morning were driven by blacks.

At one point, two black women with their children stopped their car, backed up, and asked where I was from and where I was going. After hearing my California/South Carolina song and dance, they told me, "Be careful in this warm weather," wished me good luck and drove off with women and children waving. It was a good feeling to have this rapport with them. There's hope, America!

Tired as I felt today, it was hard to get my mind off running. Yet I realized that if I did—if I disassociated—the running would go easier.

More and more, I find myself just focusing on going from one pit stop to the next. My previous focus had been on one day at a time, but nowadays even that 26-mile chunk of distance often sounds too imposing.

All told, I ran about 80 percent of today's route. Let's call it a good day, even though my ass was dragging at times.

**DAY 92.** The town where today's run started is called Cotton Plant, but a better name would be Disaster City. In all our travels, we've never seen such a dilapidated town.

There were about 15 storefronts on each side of the main street, and all were in various stages of deterioration, vandalism and abandonment. Only the post office, bank and medical clinic would pass any building inspection. We couldn't get out of town fast enough.

All along the highway today, there was a wide range in the housing from shanties to large, modern brick homes. Many of the shanties, though, had nice cars (none more than three years old) parked in front of them—Honda Accord, Buick Electra, a couple of Lincoln Continentals, a Chrysler LeBaron.

Two of the shanties were surrounded by junk. One featured six old cars, an old refrigerator, washers, tires and wheels. But it was neat compared to a shanty down the road, where the earth appeared to have vomited every conceivable type of debris.

In nearby Brinkley, I encountered the fallout from its location near Interstate 40: motels, restaurants, gas stations, fast-food places. As I moved towards the business section of Brinkley, it became apparent that this city of 800-plus souls had no zoning laws—businesses and all types of residences were interspersed through out the downtown section.

Moving through town was an interesting diversion but also a pain, because if I tried to run on the two-lane road I had to dodge oncoming cars. If I tried to run on the torn and disjointed sidewalk, I was likely to trip and trigger an injury. These were the worst running conditions of the day.

My start today was shaky. My left foot and both knees were rebelling, and it took half an hour of jog/shuffle/walk to get them into fluid operation.

Earlier, when I went by the Cache Bayou which resembles a Louisiana swamp, I had threatened some of these component body parts that if they did not get with the program, I'd jettison them in the bayou! Things got better after that.

Sort of daydreaming, I found myself thinking about the reaction of people who learn about our RUNXUSA. Their first question is almost invariably, "Why?"

I've already spelled out the reasons why. But I haven't said "Why NOT?"

People are sure we're doing it for money—money for us or for charity. Wrong, 100-percent wrong. It's costing us about $45 a day, but never have we invested more profitably.

**DAY 93.** A bit of excitement today because we would finish about 10 miles from the Mississippi River. We intended to reconnoiter the bridge that would take us out of Arkansas.

As we started at 5:20 a.m., the sky was filled with ominous clouds. The chance of rain was pegged at 50 percent. A little later, a downpour of cold rain descended on me. It had two good aspects: It was refreshing, and it drove away the mosquitoes.

Elaine, coming out for her morning jog, was caught in the same downpour. She thought that it felt wonderful.

Later, Elaine reminded me that I was still on turtle-patrol duty. I told her, "It's a real test of love when I wade through weeds and grass to scout out muddy ponds for them."

After 60 miles of scouting, I finally spotted a turtle—just the right size and on the highway. But as I came up to him I could see the poor guy had been done in by an automobile.

A bit farther along, I saw six turtles sitting on a log in a bayou. But they were too big for Elaine's specifications. Besides, I wouldn't wander out into that bayou crud for a fortune. I don't mean out swimming; I mean out even in a rowboat!

Yesterday was unique in that we didn't pass through any town. Today, took us through Marvell. Marvell High School looked to be about 35 percent gymnasium, 35 percent academic and 30 percent shops. I got the impression this would not be a good prep school for Harvard or Stanford.

This Sunday morning, I passed two churches. The United Methodist was playing to a bigger audience than the Church of Christ.

The city swimming pool was unoccupied. If I'd had a choice between the churches and the pool this warm morning, I know where I would have been.

A wild thought about running across the USA came to mind today. Maybe the ideal way to do it, since it's a once-in-a-lifetime adventure, would be to zigzag through all 48 contiguous states.

I'd estimate that seeing a representative part of each state would require 4000 miles. It could be done.

At the rate I'm running, the extra 800 miles beyond what I'm doing would take another 31 days. Another month. Thank God I didn't get that idea when planning this trek!

When suffering along in heat and humidity, as I did today, I sometimes think of a saint who was being roasted to death. It was Ignatius Loyola, if I recall correctly.

After cooking for a while, he told his executioners, "I think I'm done on this side. You'd better turn me over." Or so the story goes.

Near day's end, I asked Elaine, "When do you think I'm going to crack?" She replied, "I think you are about 2000 miles late with the question."

# E S S A Y

## *The Friend*

*(Asked to give thumbnail impressions of me, here is what several of my running friends had to say. — Paul Reese.)*

RAY MAHANNAH (a runner for more than 60 of his 76 years and co-director of the Slice 100-K): Paul is the consummate race director. The secret: The runner is paramount, first, last and always.

RUTH ANDERSON (a pioneer in women's distance running and a member of the Road Runners Club of America Hall of Fame): Paul's concern and compassion for the older athlete, and for women of all ages who finished with me at our first Pepsi 20-mile in 1973, made a lasting impression. His 50-miler in the Sacramento area in 1977 launched me into ultrarunning. But I admire him even more for fighting back from injuries and illness to continue enjoying participating. His run across the USA is a real tribute to this wonderful spirit of his.

MAVIS LINDGREN (runner of more than 60 marathons since her 70th birthday, including one at 85): I first met Paul at the Pepsi 20-Mile Run where I was doing my first long-distance run at age 69. I found him a very solicitous friend of all the runners. He and his wife Elaine were loved and admired by everyone.

ABE UNDERWOOD (veteran of the Western States 100-Mile Run and a former national masters champion at 50 miles): From the first time I saw Paul running around a park in Sacramento more than 20 years ago, he has inspired me to do things that I'd thought were well beyond my capabilities—like being a race director or running a 100-mile race. That has always been Paul's style, to set the standard for others to follow. A person's capacity can only be determined when it's tested to the limit. Paul put a lot of us to the test, and I'll never forget him for it.

LINDA ELAM (one of the few athletes to complete the Death Valley to Mount Whitney run): Besides his great-looking legs that I've only seen from behind, Paul is the true spirit of ultrarunning. Not only does he support and promote our sport, but he has the unique ability to make every runner believe in himself or herself.

PATT GALVAN (frequently competes in ultra races and finishes high in the women's masters division): Paul has been an inspiration to me as well as many others. Even with the talent he has in running, he has given encouragement to many of us with less speed.

JOAN BUMPUS (a member of the 1989 Transcontinental Relay Team): With the help of Hal Stainbrook and Ray Mahannah, Paul puts on the best races: with roller-coaster courses barren of any flatlands, with every mile marked even in the remotest locations, and with all the goodies he gives you for a token entry fee, you feel that his races cost him more than just time and effort.

JOANN HULL (a Western States 100-Mile finisher and director of the Modesto Marathon): Not only is Paul a dedicated runner, but he is also dedicated to the sport as a whole, keeping it alive by sponsoring and organizing events. He is truly an inspiration to me, and he has been since the day I met him.

STUART HONSE (a former neighbor who ran the Carson City to Sacramento race that I promoted): In our association that dates back to the early 1970s, I've contradicted Paul only once. That was as a result of a profile on him in *Ultrarunning* magazine. The interviewer asked Paul to describe his best physical feature, and his reply was, "My sexy legs." Whereupon I was prompted to write to the magazine and state, "Only Elaine would consider his bird-legs sexy."

JAN LEVET (has completed more than 50 ultramarathons): All told, I've run in 10 of Paul's races. From those experiences, I quickly learned to respect his aplomb, his directness and his ability to get quickly to the meat of the task at hand. Paul takes risks, and that's what makes him free.

SALLY EDWARDS (founder and president of Fleet Feet Inc., author of eight books and masters record-holder in the Ironman Triathlon): Paul is a man of many missions. He is a runner; hence this story. He is an educator; hence this book. He is a husband-father; hence his perspective that his children and grandchildren and their friends will read this book and know that they, too, can accomplish something extraordinary if they set their mind to it.

RALPH PAFFENBARGER (my companion in hundreds of racing miles): Paul Francis Reese is very special to the hundreds of us who call ourselves long-distance runners. We admire not only his personal physical accomplishments, but also his scholarly academic contributions to health and fitness. He has given us sound and explicit advice on how to put zest into living. And by personal example, as narrated in this volume, he has exemplified the true meanings of dedication, determination and discipline.

# Overview of Mississippi

## July 23 to 30, 1990 — 178.3 miles — 2601.4 total

| Day | Overnight | Miles | Notes |
|-----|-----------|-------|-------|
| 94 | Sardis | 26.4 | last 5.0 miles in Mississippi |
| 95 | near Sardis | 26.4 | |
| 96 | Sardis Lake | 26.2 | |
| 97 | near Galena | 26.3 | completed 2500 miles, temperature hit 101 degrees |
| 98 | New Albany | 26.3 | |
| 99 | Tupelo | 26.7 | |
| 100 | near Dennis | 26.4 | |

(first 15.2 miles in Mississippi on Day 101)

## Chapter 9

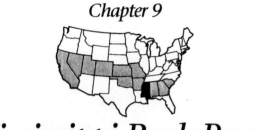

# *Mississippi Back Roads*

Most Americans carry a mental picture of the Mississippi River splitting the country down the middle. Not so. On crossing this mighty river, we would have completed almost three-fourths of our journey east. Less than 800 miles remained.

The countdown was tilting heavily in our favor as we entered Mississippi to run 178 miles between July 23 and July 30. Eight states in the bank, four to go.

**DAY 94.** After yesterday's finish, we rushed to the Mississippi River for a reconnaissance. We learned to our dismay that a construction project had restricted part of the bridge to one lane, and traffic on that portion was controlled by a stoplight.

The bridge also had no sidewalk or breakdown lane. But I was so excited about crossing the Mississippi that those shortcomings didn't dampen my enthusiasm.

We started this landmark day short on sleep. Unable to find an RV hookup, we'd parked overnight at the Arkansas Tourist Information Center.

The motor home stayed uncomfortably hot until around 11 p.m., when a breeze began to stir. A heavy downpour followed.

Much of the evening, we had entertainment provided by a black pimp and his two white prostitutes. The pimp watched the alcohol-primed women from a parked car. Their M.O. was to approach the male drivers who stopped to use the restroom.

I stepped out of the motor home this morning to see a sky full of nasty clouds. Rain fell heavily within a few miles, and Elaine got caught in it for the second time in two days during her morning jog.

Running from mile four to 11 in the rain, I was reminded

that it's easier in this part of the country to run in the refreshing rain than in the humid heat. One trick I use in this rainy weather is to rub Aspercreme on my legs. It sheds water and, to a degree, keeps the legs warm.

As we approached the Mississippi bridge, Elaine called the Helena police to tell them about what time I'd be running across. We had corresponded with them when planning the route, and they'd replied, "The bridge is under construction and we don't want pedestrians crossing it, but we'll make exceptions for valid reasons."

In my case, they said, they would provide an escort. I asked Elaine to tell them if they were busy, I was confident—based on yesterday's recon—that I could across the bridge safely.

Elaine returned with a newspaper reporter, Marla Clark, in tow. Marla had heard about our run from the Tourist Information Center and had interviewed Elaine when she stopped there to make her call. The reporter, a graduate of the University of Arkansas journalism school, was an attractive young lady with a drawl you could trip over.

Elaine told me, "The police are tied up in court and might not be able to provide the escort. If they don't appear, you're to negotiate the bridge by yourself."

Arriving at the bridge, I saw no police. Seeing no cars approaching from the left lane, I busted my butt running the hill and got two-thirds of the way up before the first cars appeared.

I stopped, hugged the bridge rail and waited until they passed. I ran again until reaching a 12-inch ledge—almost a sidewalk—that ran the length of the center span.

I then ran on the road whenever possible and jumped to the ledge as cars drew close. Standing there on one such occasion and watching the river go by, I was treated to the sight of a huge, loaded barge passing beneath the bridge.

After the last car went through the stoplight at the end of the bridge, I took off as fast as I could before the light turned loose another flock of cars. I knew damn well that this all-out effort would cost me dearly as the miles mounted later in the day. But I was triumphant, reaching the highway just as the first car started up the bridge.

Elaine's crossing was nerve-wracking, too, because the one lane on the bridge was barely wide enough to accommodate the motor home. Considering the problem of crossing the Mississippi on foot, we were lucky in our choice of route, because no Interstate highways lead to or from this bridge, and approaching and exiting it was relatively simple.

A few miles into Mississippi, I ran out of zip. Couldn't decide whether this resulted from the restless night or from sprinting across the bridge.

The sense of progress at entering a new state can't override the feeling that this day has been sort of a downer.

**DAY 95.** After a comfortable night in Sardis, we drove 29 miles to the start this morning. This was the longest interval yet from our overnight spot.

First question on my mind, as I hit the road today was, "How hungry are the mosquitoes?" Bravely, I set forth without any protective Off.

I baptized another new pair of shoes—my sixth—this morning. I'm still sticking exclusively with the New Balance 840s.

Love the dogs in this part of the country. Most of them are on the porch or near the house. Seeing me, they give a bark or two, then with an attitude of, "The hell with it; I've done my duty," they return to resting.

I stopped to scout several ponds for turtles today, but no sightings. One thing I did see as I looked down from bridges was that the people hereabouts dump much garbage into the creeks and rivers.

Sociological note: All through Kansas, Missouri, Oklahoma, Arkansas and now Mississippi, I've seen laundry on clotheslines. That is rarely seen these days in California.

At an early pit stop, Elaine noted the negative way that folks here ask questions. She'd had two offers of help when parked here. The exact words were, "Y'all aren't broken down, are you?" and, "Y'all don't need any help, do you?"

I got a sample when a fellow asked, "You ain't in trouble, are you?"

A short while later, a farmer—white, knowledgeable, and most likely prosperous—stopped to talk with me and explained the cotton process. Cotton harvesting, I learned, takes place around October.

I asked him if there was any flooding in this delta area. He said, "It's somewhat common, but watersheds prevent major flooding."

A young driver pulled up alongside me, told me he'd seen me in Helena, and wanted to know, "Are you running across the country?" He drove alongside me for half a mile as I reported on the run. His curiosity satisfied, he wished me good luck and took off.

Then a couple of friendly black farmers, curious about what I was doing out here, stopped their pickup to talk with me. After I told them, I suspected they were questioning my sanity.

All this visiting today was enjoyable. It slowed my progress, but one of the reasons we are in the back country is to meet the people.

I did a bit of disassociating by thinking about the cruise Elaine wants to take when we finish this safari. On the road like this, planning for a cruise is damn difficult. Since Elaine mentioned this possibility three weeks ago, we have not gone through one town that has a travel agency in it.

So I've had to write to California for cruise information. Now the next trick will be for that info to arrive at one of our general delivery post office addresses.

Much as I am enjoying this cross-country trek, if after I reach the Atlantic someone were to say, "Now I'll give you $100,000 to reverse course and run back to the Pacific," I'd refuse the offer. Definitely.

**DAY 96.** When we went through Sardis yesterday on our way to overnighting at John Kyle State Park, I stopped for a haircut. Doing so in this small town reminded me of a scene in *Treasure of the Sierra Madre*, in which Humphrey Bogart goes into a barber shop in a small Mexican town and comes out with a weird haircut.

"Will I meet the same fate in Sardis?" I wondered. First surprise, the barber was a woman. Second surprise, outstanding haircut. Some days you just live right!

"Oh God, if only I could stay in bed," I thought while forcing myself out at 4:30 a.m. to face another day of 26-plus miles. Our day didn't begin joyously. When Elaine and I went out to unplug the electrical and water hookups, we were caught in a blizzard of mosquitoes.

I've battled mosquitoes in Alaska, the Solomon Islands and North Carolina. But never had so many hit us as this morning.

The approach to Sardis this morning was scenic—two miles or more of road lined with pine trees on each side. Too bad so much litter detracted from this beauty. Mississippi has an adopt-a-highway program, but the adopters must have abandoned this child.

This was a day when I attracted almost as many curiosity-seekers as mosquitoes. It started when Elaine parked for a pit stop, met some people there and talked with them. When I came along, they were all standing there to see this 73-year-old man who runs. It has come to this!

But, wait, there were two encores. Three miles later, where Elaine again had been visiting, half a dozen folks had gathered— yes, to see this 73-year-old man who runs. We exchanged greetings and joked with each other.

Later still, Elaine had scored again. Three guys wanted, in their words, "to see what the 73-year-old wonder boy looks like."

I was beginning to feel like an oddity, especially while in the motor home enjoying a snack when these three guys returned with a friend. He opened the screen door, stuck his head in, and said, "I just got to see what you look like."

At least these men contributed to the cause. They gave us directions to a nearby RV park with a good restaurant adjacent. And of course they recommended the catfish, a standard menu item in these parts.

Though both of my knees acted up on and off during the day, I finished without laboring unduly. Fact is, the last 13 miles went better than the first 13 miles.

On my mind at the end: "Twenty-seven days to go. Hang in there, baby, and, Lord, let our good luck continue!"

Our evening hookup is at the Holiday Lodge on Sardis Lake. At dinner, Elaine went native by ordering catfish and hush puppies. My concession to the South was ordering country-fried ham. Good food, nice evening.

**DAY 97.** Surprisingly, no kinks or twitches as I took off this morning. Maybe de ole body am numb!

Of course, by now I'm battle-wise enough to know that the first half-hour is critical. That's the time to ease into the run and assess its effects. Sure enough, I was running along fine when suddenly I got a knee twitch. It reminded me how dicey my health is.

The farther I get into this run, the more tired become the muscles, tendons and bones, and the more apprehensive I become when I feel a problem come on. I'm afraid it could develop into the collapse of a working body component, and then I'll be in big trouble.

A thought keeps crossing my mind, one I can't express too often or too emphatically: On a trek like this, the runner's got to believe—believe he can keep going, believe he'll make it to the end, believe that doing this serves a worthwhile purpose.

In my 27 years of running, I've learned that one of the best fallouts of being on the road alone is the time it allows for meditation. Boy, I'm doing a lot of that out here—about on a par with a Trappist monk.

Here's an assortment of thoughts on the run, recorded as they came to me today:

* Many of the Mississippi drivers follow the practice seen ever since Colorado. Much before sun-up, they're driving without lights. I hear them before I see them.

* Along a levee road, with bayous on both sides of the road, I hear noises emanating from these swamps. A bit eerie in the darkness.

* At the five-mile pit stop, Elaine treats me to pancakes and hot syrup. Now we'll see if that fuels me. My fifth mile was laborious. Wonder why.

* Elaine comes out for her second morning jog. She reminds me that the big turtle hunt is still on.

* Coming in for the next pit stop, I tease Elaine by saying, "I saw this small turtle and I asked him, 'Do you want to go to South Carolina?' He said, 'Git away from me, skinny ol' white man!'"

* Finding Highway 7 a magnet for fast traffic, we detour to the traffic-free frontage road which parallels it. Some of this road is through bayous, some beside little streams. Fertile with turtle, I'm thinking. But all my hunting is in vain and it eats into my running time. Where can I buy a turtle? Price be damned!

* Being pestered now by some big horse flies. When I say "big," I mean about the size of a grasshopper. Funny thing about them is they buzz me all day as if coming in for a landing, but only one has bitten. By one of these guys, once is enough.

* At the last pit stop, Elaine shows me a one-inch by two-inch hole in the fiberglass screen on our motor home window. She says, "I was sitting in the dining area, heard this noise by the screen and looked up to see some huge insect gobbling the fiberglass." She doused him with Raid and patched the screen with tape. This is her excitement for the day.

* This road is a prize-winner for traffic. In 10 miles, I've seen six cars. It's been a memorable day in that there was not a single offer of help all day. Probably because I was running such a blazing pace!

We're winding down this day at Wall Doxey State Park.

Like so many parks we've seen in the South, this one is only 10-percent occupied at the height of the summer season. In California, it would be overbooked.

**DAY 98.** Out in the boondocks, amidst light fog and a fanfare of dogs, we started the day with a bit of anticipation. We'd have a mail call at New Albany.

The first town, Bethlehem, was nothing but a gathering of homes and one small grocery and gas station—plus a couple of churches, of course. I didn't see any mangers in Bethlehem, but some stars were shining brightly.

Yesterday brought not a single offer of help. But early this morning, a plasterer in a pickup stopped to ask, "You aren't having trouble, are you?"

Later, just outside of Bethlehem, I told a second fellow that we are running across the USA. He didn't seem to grasp the concept, a common problem in Mississippi.

As I made my morning assessment of aches and pains, I philosophized that if I run into trouble it will first be because of joints, second because of bones, third because of tendons and fourth because of muscles.

My left knee gave me a heap of trouble this morning. It's my biggest concern, and my right knee ranks next.

I made a deal with God today, and I hope He buys it. If my knees hold together, I promise not to bitch about the road conditions, the traffic or the heat.

All of the above were, at best, marginal today. I'm not complaining, mind you—just reporting.

My deal must have been accepted. Either God intervened, or a magic cure came in the form of Elaine's fresh peach coffee cake. After that pit stop, the knee pain eased from quite worrisome to only slightly annoying.

Today could be called "dog day." Dozens of dogs barked at me. I'm beginning to sense that there is a difference between the bark of a chained or fenced dog and a dog running loose. The restrained dog sounds more pitiful or more frantic.

Several unanswered questions about Mississippi came up during today's trek:

1. I go by church after church, most of them nice brick buildings. How can such a sparse population support so many churches?

2. In an area with so few people, I passed by a place with six large moving vans parked out front. Who (okay, WHOM) do they move?

3. Amidst generally low-quality housing, I occasionally saw what could only be described as a mansion. Why would someone who could afford to build such a home choose to put it here?

4. Throughout Mississippi, I've noticed that dumpsters are placed at various road junctions for the deposit of garbage. Why, then, are Mississippi roads strewn with more litter than any state I've seen?

A first today: A Mississippi state trooper stopped to ask, "You aren't having any trouble, are you?" He was a black officer, very professional and built like an All-American tackle.

Score one for Mississippi. We didn't get that kind of concern in other recent states.

My thoughts today gravitated to August, just four days away. Rounding the corner into that month will put us on the home stretch, and that will be a morale booster.

Funny, as I go along, how I put these things into chapters. Months, states. Little bites to chew on.

**DAY 99.** We ended yesterday by a cemetery on the east end of New Albany. Rather than drive 25 miles to the nearest RV park, we settled for a motel. The price was right—a room with a king-sized bed for $29.95 at the Hallmark Inn.

It was sheer torture for Elaine and me to exit that bed shortly after four a.m. Our day began a bit differently because we went to a restaurant and had waffles for breakfast before launching the run.

The starting surroundings were none too cheerful—a cemetery on one side of us and a funeral home on the other.

Just as Elaine drove off, a black cat ran in front of the motor home. Almost immediately, we ran into misfortune. We came to an unmarked intersection and in the dark took the wrong road, wasting seven-tenths of a mile.

Again this morning, my left knee wasn't with the program. Also, I realized that 10 minutes after eating a waffle and drinking three cups of coffee is not the smartest time to start running. Burp, burp!

As I reached down to the depths today for energy and drive, I reminded myself, "We are enjoying!"

I'm learning that while I have to assess and humor an injury, like this knee today, at the same time I can't let it overwhelm me. I've got to be aggressive—assume an attitude of, "Damn the injuries. Full speed ahead." (Thank you, Admiral Farragut, for the paraphrase.)

There has been nothing unusually scenic or exciting today, so I think I'll dub this "appreciation day." I started out wondering, "Lord, if the left knee acts this way after I've had eight hours of sleep, what's it going to do after 15 or more miles on the road?" Somehow the knee rehabilitated itself and I was able to run 85 to 90 percent of today's route. I appreciate!

While running, I reflected on a letter received yesterday from my daughter Susan. We'd asked her for help with cruise planning because none of the last 30 towns we passed through had a travel agency.

Susie reported that all the Bermuda cruises are seven days, while the most Elaine and I want is five. So that eliminates Bermuda. Seems our next-best bet is to check on four- or five-day cruises to the Virgin Islands or Caribbean.

Yeah, I'm still on turtle patrol. During the last couple of days, I've scouted 30 or more ponds and creeks and not spotted a single turtle. I'm inclined to add, "and not a married one either." This running is getting to me!

The workday done, we drove 24 miles to Elvis Presley State Park near Elvis' birthplace. This evening, Elaine played her guitar which, no doubt, had The King rolling over in his grave.

**DAY 100.** A frustrating and infuriating day on the road. It started with having to wait for a ranger (shoeless and dressed only in ball cap and swim trunks) to open the gate at Elvis Presley State Park.

After the 27-mile drive from the park to our start, then another 10 miles of road reconnaissance, plus the hard running of yesterday, I had trouble getting in gear this morning. I was, to put it mildly, not Gung Ho.

The plan was to follow back roads today. But our planning didn't account for the fact that most of these roads would be unmarked.

We had to depend on the locals for navigation. The first help came from a high school kid out skateboarding.

A little later, I spotted a fellow savoring his morning cup of coffee out in front of his mobile home. I stopped to pump him for some backroad information.

On the dusty trunk of his car, he drew a map showing how to reach Highway 4. I memorized his map and shoved off, only to find this one of the trickiest courses we've yet negotiated.

Every so often, I had to find somebody to confirm that I was headed the right way. Or I should say, Elaine usually found somebody, then relayed the word to me. Getting these directions often required flagging down a car.

Kind of strange to be going through a small community of 100 homes and not even know where I am. But our navigation proved successful, as we eventually reached Highway 4.

Now I knew where I was but didn't care to be there. This road featured most of what I hate about highways, being narrow, busy, curvy and slanted.

This entire stretch of road was lined with homes, never more than a quarter-mile apart and usually clustered closer. Ninety-eight percent of them were residential (as opposed to farmhouses).

What mystified me was how those 98 percent of homeowners earn their living. What businesses, what industries support them? Lord knows there was no visible means of support out here.

Most of the drivers were courteous, but I'm discovering they don't waste energy here in the South. A guy will have all 10 of his fingers wrapped around the steering wheel of his pickup. When he waves, he'll lift only his index finger.

Two incidents occurred on Highway 4 that still make me furious as I write about them. First, I saw this car coming fast down the hill, so I moved a couple of feet out onto the gravel shoulder. No other cars were on the road. But this guy swerved over to the gravel shoulder and headed straight for me.

At first, I didn't believe it. Then, realizing it was truly happening, I jumped out farther. He swerved back to the highway at the last possible moment, and I saw the driver and his two passengers laughing as they went by. Lucky I wasn't packing a gun.

Near the finish, four teenagers in the back of a pickup threw some type of firecracker toward me and enjoyed seeing me jump. Demonstrating superb restraint, I didn't salute them with an obscene gesture.

Can't remember how long it's been since I've had this tough a day. I just plain dragged ass the whole way.

I've heard pilots say, "Any landing you can walk from is a good landing." I guess a transcon runner can say, "Any day you can walk away from without a sustained injury is a good day." By that token, this day was okay.

We've now completed 100 days on the road without missing a single takeoff or landing. The celebrating will come tomorrow when we enter Alabama.

# E S S A Y

## The Explorer
by Theresa McCourt

*(Theresa McCourt is the running columnist for the* Sacramento Bee, *a position I once held. She's quite a runner in her own right with a personal best for the marathon of 2:50:11 and for the 10-K, 36:59. —Paul Reese.)*

It is tempting to measure ourselves by numbers, and Paul Reese has them: more than 50 ultramarathons and 225 marathons, plus age-group records by the bushel.

But Paul is not humbugged into measuring himself this way. He runs for experiences, not statistics.

Stats are dry, one-dimensional. Experience is rich, dense, multi-layered.

To run for stats is to burn out. To run for experience is to enjoy and endure, as Paul has done.

He did not run across the USA because of an immature fight to recapture his youth and manhood. He did it to heighten his senses to the possibilities of old age.

"People have missed the whole point if they see it as a jock thing," he says. "Running through the South, I saw a lot of older folks sitting on their front porches in rocking chairs, watching the world go by.

"To me, that's not quality of life. This trip was."

Paul ran across America to see the country in slow motion, to take the back roads, to FEEL the sun rise and set over the deserts and mountains. He took this journey not just to engage life but to celebrate it wholeheartedly.

Only three years before, he continued running while being treated for prostate cancer. There are several ways to perceive someone who runs through cancer.

Perhaps denial, perhaps anger. Or perhaps Paul's simple way of accepting adversity was as he would luck—as nothing personal, just doing the best he can no matter what the limitations.

"It wasn't to say, 'Look at me, Mr. Genes, Mr. Macho,'" he says of that experience. "I didn't want to come off like, 'Boy, I had cancer and I'm a tiger right now.'"

Instead, Paul speaks modestly. He recognizes the part chance played in his fate.

"I was just lucky that my cancer was detected early," he says. "It hadn't metastasized. The early detection and my recovery are a tribute to modern medicine, not running."

Whenever Paul talks of his accomplishments, he tries to distract us from perceptions of himself as someone out of the ordinary. Though his times may rank him higher than others, he sees such rankings as the false gods of running. What he cares for most is the inner effect of his best and most enduring efforts, not the outward scoring.

He insists that each of us has this same ability to make the most of our lives. He wants us to recognize that we can weave our distinct self into the complex and sometimes overwhelming scheme of life.

This self, he says, deserves a voice. Running is only one of many ways to help it speak.

# Overview of Alabama

### July 30 to August 6, 1990 — 181.7 miles — 2783.1 total

| Day | Overnight | Miles | Notes |
| --- | --- | --- | --- |
| 101 | Halltown | 26.2 | last 11.0 miles in Alabama |
| 102 | Russellville | 26.5 | temperature hit 100 degrees |
| 103 | Hartselle | 26.5 | |
| 104 | Decatur | 26.3 | |
| 105 | Guntersville | 26.6 | |
| 106 | near Oak Grove | 26.2 | |
| 107 | Fort Payne | 26.2 | |

(first 12.4 miles in Alabama on Day 108)

*Chapter 10*

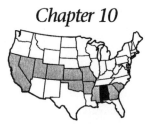

# Into August in Alabama

Alabama in August. Those words had a nice ring to them for reasons other than alliteration.

Entering Alabama would put us one state closer to our finish line. Moving into August would put us into the final month of our trek that had begun way back in April.

Alabama would still be the sultry South, though. August would be the depths of summer as we trudged the 181 miles scheduled from July 30 to August 6.

**DAY 101.** We drove to our start brimming with good cheer. Elaine had whipped up a spaghetti dinner last night. That's great body fuel, so I was counting on moving a bit today.

We savored our early morning drive on the Natchez Trace Parkway, a road where commercial vehicles are prohibited. The Trace extends from Tishomingo State Park on the north all the way across the Mississippi to Natchez on the south.

Unfortunately, we only got to drive this dream-road. The running roads were more mundane, but they would lead us into Alabama this morning.

We hit the Mississippi-Alabama border at the west city limit of Red Bay. It's so-named, I assume, because the soil in this area is the same type of red clay that I've seen in places as diverse as Georgia, Guam and Placerville, California.

The approach to most of the small towns we've seen has been through a corridor of residences. Not so with Red Bay. We were into heavy business development immediately. From all the action, including an Allegro motor home plant, I surmised that the local economy is good.

Shortly after entering town, I came upon a windfall. The

road had a three-foot paved breakdown lane. Yea, 'Bama!

This was another of those mornings when the air was clean, the traffic light, the air cool. Again, I found myself wishing I'd been out here half an hour or more earlier.

That would have meant spending that much less time out in the thunderstorm and heavy rain which were with me the last five or six miles this afternoon. Actually, through, being wet isn't as uncomfortable as being hot. But the major problem with rain is the damage it does to shoes. I'm wearing the last pair we have onboard, and a new pair won't arrive until we pick up mail in Guntersville five days from now.

It took me a while to notice that something was missing in the last few miles today. Unlike Arkansas and Mississippi which had houses at least every quarter-mile, there were none along this nine-mile stretch in Alabama.

As I go along, it becomes increasingly evident that I'm not recovering overnight as well as I did a month or so ago. I'm trying to take one day at a time and am relieved every day I finish without a debilitating injury. At the same time, I'm apprehensive about being able to continue without getting hurt.

Strength comes just from knowing when the trek will be over. I've done more calculating and now figure that we should finish August 22.

**DAY 102.** A scary beginning to our morning at Bear Creek Reservoir Campground. We were up shortly after 4:00 a.m. and at 4:20 heard a knock on the motor home door.

"Yes," I called. Two more knocks in the predawn darkness.

"What do you want?" I shouted. Hesitation, then, "I have a memorandum for you from the camp commander."

This sounded phony. First, the camp manager had told us yesterday all we needed to know. Second, what reasonable person would be sending us a memo at four o'clock in the morning?

I replied, "We don't need it," and waited for the knocker's next move. "OK," he said, then walked to his car and drove off.

After he left, I was sorry not to have turned on the motor home porch light to get a look at the man and not to have checked the make of car. Two lessons learned.

A few minutes later, as we exited the motor home to unhook our water and electrical connections, we were on full alert. And as we drove out to Highway 24, we remained wary of what we might find on the way. One plus about this kind of action: It pumps the adrenaline.

Our further encounters with people were all pleasant today, as it turned out. An elderly gent, wearing an oversize cowboy hat and speaking with a rich Alabama drawl, stopped to ask, "What's goin' on?"

Elaine, with me on her morning jog, explained the situation. Besides being pilot, navigator and cook, she has taken on public relations duties.

I've noticed that most of the Alabama men drivers wave when they spot me. The women don't. They're paralyzed with the thought, "What's this old coot doing out here in his BVDs?"

After 26 miles in Alabama, I finally saw my first state trooper and first black person. They were one and the same, and he asked, "Are you just out for exercise?" I explained the task at hand and what our M.O. is. Then we had an enjoyable 15-minute conversation.

The trooper was a bright young man with a degree in business administration. "Before joining the Highway Patrol," he said, "I worked in an office but didn't like the confinement. I like the work I'm doing now because it gets me out and lets me meet people."

I asked him a number of questions. For example, "Why don't we see any deer?"

He told me that they mostly stay way from this highway. "But in a four-mile stretch of the area we're on now, cars recently have hit a total of eight deer, causing injuries to people and damage to cars—not to mention fatalities to the deer."

I also asked him about snakes in Alabama. The trooper said, "Rattlers, copperheads and water moccasins are about." Just the kind of news I needed.

During the 15 minutes we talked, we were within sight of Elaine as she waited for me in the motor home. When I joined her, she asked, "Was he telling you not to run on this road?" She was greatly relieved to hear what we really were discussing.

Talking with this state trooper turned out to be the highlight of my running day. Another good aspect was that it brought down the curtain on July. Tomorrow begins the final act.

After finishing today, we couldn't find an RV park within 20 miles. So we decided to drive to Russellville and tap our motel budget to the tune of $31.50 at the Village Inn.

Now in the spending mood, we dined—maybe not elegantly but at least enjoyably—at the Pizza Hut. Hey, that Veggie Lover's pan pizza was ammunition for tomorrow's run!

**DAY 103.** Hello, August! Never before have I been so glad to see you. Now we're on the homestretch.

We got an early start, five a.m. to be precise. This usually is the best time of day for running, but for the first time an early start disappointed us.

The traffic—mainly from trucks—was furious, and there was no shoulder for my running or for Elaine to pull off and park. We were anything but simmering with enthusiasm.

The main danger on this road was that many 14-foot-wide mobile homes were being towed. I measured the road and found it to be not quite 11 feet from the white fog line to the center line of the road. Uh, oh!

In just two hours this morning, I counted 10 of these oversized mobile homes on the road. They're manufactured in nearby Red Bay, Alabama, by Sunshine Homes. This same outfit makes Sunshine cat and dog food. If there's a connection there, it's lost on me.

These homes were preceded by a pilot car with flashing lights, and this was one time when I saw trucks move to the far side of the road to give the oversized homes road space. Not for a minute on this road could I take my mind off traffic, since I have this burning desire to survive.

During Elaine's morning jog with me, we were running against traffic when we got a scare. A hare-brained woman in a Cadillac, passing a truck and seeing us only as she was upon us, came within six inches of hitting us. A goose-pimple experience.

For the first time since we started in April, I've taken out the New Balance 840 inserts and in their place put Spenco orthotics. This big experiment happened by accident.

I tested the inserts last night and in my early morning confusion forgot to switch back to the regular inserts. Going along, it suddenly occurred to me that I was running with the Spencos. I think they helped, just as they once had in the Western States 100.

We've been trying to buy beer the past couple of days. Not the hard stuff, mind you, but the non-alcoholic variety. We've struck out and finally learned why. In Alabama, counties control alcohol sales and the last two counties we've passed through are dry. This ban covers Sharp's, O'Doul's and the like because they contain a tiny amount of alcohol.

Arriving in the town of Moulton, our long search for a travel agency finally ended. Elaine picked up the cruise brochures we'd been hoping to find.

At our next pit stop, I glanced at the brochures as fuel for disassociating by doing some cruise planning. I needed to get my mind on something else besides the miles when they begin to hang heavily, as they did today.

Other than moving into August, there was no particular excitement or highlight to this day. Well, I guess you could say that escaping Highway 24 unscathed was reason for celebration.

We drove into Hartselle to scout for an RV hookup, found none and decided to live dangerously—and economically. We're parked for the night in a shopping center lot.

**DAY 104.** I started the day relieved that we had no problems sleeping last night while parked at the shopping center. Sans air conditioning, though, the motor home was warm.

The morning body assessment showed my left foot to be a bit gimpy and my left quad to be strained. I need a left leg transplant.

However, my legs felt spunky when I finished yesterday. Could have been the Spenco orthotics that I baptized then, so I tried them again today.

Today's outstanding town was Hartselle. It definitely had personality. Its four-block business section had a metal awning covering all the store fronts, making this sort of an outdoor mall. The wrought iron decorating the awning reflects history.

At our first pit stop, Elaine had parked at the entrance to a lovely brick home—probably a $400,000 value in California. But what caught my eye was the magnificent, lofty, symmetrical tree—an oak, I believe—in the front yard.

It was the most beautiful tree I've seen on this trip. Joyce Kilmer must have been looking at one like this when he wrote "Trees." Driving, I would not have noticed it.

Later, we passed by another elegant Alabama home. It sat 100 yards off the road and had a front yard the size of a football field. The two-story brick house had at least 10 rooms. Like many homes in this area, it flew a flag—U.S., not Confederate, as I would have expected.

The only substandard housing was in Danville. Judging from the metal bars I saw on home and store windows, Danville didn't appear to be the finest of communities.

One thing I've not mentioned about Southern homes. In Missouri, Arkansas, Mississippi and now Alabama, about 80 percent of them have a couple of chairs on the front porch, and some also have a swing.

Yesterday I thought the Burn Out Baptist Church and the Highway 36 Baptist Church were the most unusual names I'd seen. But how about this one today: Ironman Baptist Church.

Road-survival lesson for the day: I've got to remember to turn my back when logging and gravel trucks go by. Bark or gravel falls off and hits me, and that could be an eye-closer.

There is some large-scale farming in this area, and the farmers must be doing well. They all have large brick homes.

I entertained myself this morning by watching a farmer with a tractor pulling a cutter/thresher. The machine cut a row of corn stalks, picked them up and deposited them in a mulcher, which then dumped them in a truck for use as cattle feed.

As the miles added up, I mulled over which leg of each day's run is the toughest. It's a tossup between miles 17-20 and 20-23. Miles 23-26 don't match the earlier ones for toughness because they're softened by my knowing that the end is near.

Today, I saw the sun only on the 23-26 leg. Rain traveled with me the rest of the way, and I loved the refreshing coolness of it. Heat and humidity enervate me more than mileage.

We're hooked up for the night at Point Mallard Campground in Decatur. The centerpiece of this 750-acre park is America's first wave pool (or so they advertise).

The facility also features an Olympic-sized pool, a miniature golf course, an 18-hour championship golf course and an ice rink—none of which we tested. Running water and air conditioning provided all the entertainment we needed.

**DAY 105.** This started as a day of anticipation for Elaine and me. We would get our only Alabama mail, this in Guntersville.

We were supposed to get brochures to help with our cruise planning. We were also expecting info to help us decide on our finish area. This has come down to a choice between two spots in South Carolina—the Marine Corps Air Station at Beaufort or Hilton Head Island.

Elaine and I have noticed that Alabama seems to reflect more affluence than Mississippi. Also, prices are higher here.

Most of the homes along today's route were farmhouses. I'd estimate that about 45 percent of these were middle-class, 45 percent were modest homes, and 10 percent were homes that would cost $300,000 in California.

For some reason, even though we were on a county road among farms, I got the impression of suburbia rather than a farming belt. For many of these people, farming appeared to be avocational.

Much of my route ran along narrow, hilly, winding roads through the backcountry. Marring the beauty of this forested area was a trail of litter.

An official highway sign I saw today was more blunt than any I've encountered in 2500 miles. It read: "Slow. Dead Man's Curve. Dangerous."

This sign also portrayed accurately the bad aspects of today's hills. They can be dangerous, and they slowed my running. But on the positive side, I suspect the ups and downs are somewhat therapeutic as compared to the constant flats.

Much as I am enjoying the overall experience of this transcon run, there are times that are downers—like when I came out of the motor home after the 13-mile pit stop today.

I was thinking, "I'm tired, sluggish, hot. And I have to do this all over again, another 13 miles. How in hell am I able to do it?" I shuddered at the thought, then reminded myself, "Just have to hang in there like a marathoner hangs in for the late miles. Just keep moving forward until the job is done."

I must admit to a double-barreled piece of stupidity today. Forgot to fill my water bottle for the 16- to 19-mile leg. Then to show that I'm a slow learner, I repeated that act for the 19-22 leg.

The scene changed abruptly as we reached Highway 69, a heavily traveled four-lane road leading into Guntersville. The long drop down into town offered the most picturesque scene of the day. Heavy forest growth bracketed both sides of the road, and straight ahead to the east lay a dam and the Tennessee River. Not a bad way to end a day.

We drove into Guntersville for our mail, and here we got an unexpected bonus. Along with cruise brochures from my daughter Susan came some Sacramento newspapers from my son Mark.

But there were also minuses. The expected shoes didn't arrive, nor did any replies from Beaufort or Hilton Head to our inquiries about finishing there.

**DAY 106.** Elaine and I were up late last night doing cruise planning. This lack of sleep made the running a chore today, and now it's influencing my ability to write coherently.

I'm ready for another as-it-happened report. Tape recorder, do your duty:

Instead of starting in the boondocks as usual, we're on the outskirts of Guntersville. The highway is four lanes, and we're lucky to be getting through town before its annual festival begins today.

It's misty and invigorating as I start. After a mile, I reach a lake with a causeway bisecting it and see a marina with 200 to 300 boats.

I come upon a crane standing on a rock by the lake, and it takes off as I come near. It skims over the water. Never before have I been able to look down on a flying crane like this, and it has a beautiful flight pattern.

Thirty ducks nearby swim farther out into the lake. In the distant east, I see heavily forested mountains.

As I cross the causeway bridge, I notice a huge spider web about every foot, which prompts me to move out into the road more. The traffic being almost non-existent, I stop smack in the middle of the causeway to get rid of some coffee.

At the east edge of the causeway, I see that the city has an attractive recreational complex bordered by lake and forest. There's an air of adventure and excitement when I go along seeing new and different scenery instead of farm after farm.

Not that some of the farming hasn't been entertaining to watch—the wheat harvesting, the corn threshing and mulching, the spray coupes in action, the sophisticated machinery. I'm getting the impression that a successful farmer is somewhat of a scientist.

The day is heating up as the thought hits me: If a guy is not adaptable to heat, the odds are against him ever finishing a transcontinental run.

I'm now on Highway 75. For running, it's the pits. As has happened so regularly across the country, a driver will have the entire road to himself but won't give me any running space. I think this results more from a lack of thinking than a lack of courtesy.

Yet at times some old geezer will bear down on me, and his attitude is readable: "What the hell are you doing running on MY road!"

Here's what I call chimpanzee mentality: I'm running along with no traffic coming toward me. A car approaches from behind, and the driver crosses the yellow line to my side and yells to startle me.

What he doesn't know is that I'm too tired to react. That has been my problem today—tired, drained of energy.

Finally, we reach Geraldine. How's that for a town name? Imagine if it has a high school and the cheerleaders yell, "Rah, rah, go, Geraldine!"

We finish our day near this town on Highway 75. This leaves me with the unhappy thought that I've got to run this snakepit road again tomorrow.

My evening's map work reveals that we have 475 miles left. We can make that in 18 days. Ah yes, the countdown is definitely on.

**DAY 107.** Even recalling Guadalcanal and the Solomon Islands, I can't remember it being as hot and humid in the morning as it is in Alabama. I felt about as tired in the early miles today as I usually do at the 23-mile mark.

Then at a pit stop, I read a newspaper clipping my son Mark had sent me about a 60-year-old friend of mine who had died of a heart attack. I resumed running with the thought, "Hey, I'm not so tired after all. I'm lucky just to be out here at my age."

Later, I caught myself serenading a herd of cows as they lingered around a pond. The song? "Dixie," of course. These cows were among the few living creatures that would listen to my singing. Compared to me, George Burns is Caruso.

Bad day for dogs. I passed a young Collie, newly killed on the highway. Then, on her morning jog, Elaine moved a recently departed Shepherd pup from the road to keep it from being hamburgered by the cars.

At Rainsville, I called my daughter Susan who has been handling our household business. I gave her some guidelines for a four-night cruise to the Bahamas, and invited her and husband Ed to accompany us. Now it's Susie's job to make all the arrangements.

Excitement prevaileth! Cruise, cruise, cruise!

Susie also relayed a message from some Marine Corps classmates in Georgia. They want to visit us on the road and welcome us to Georgia.

Highway 35 from Rainsville to Fort Payne was bumper-to-bumper housing. Some homes were residential and some sat on farms so small they could be called "backyard" farms.

Nearing Fort Payne, I went down a long, steep hill on a road so narrow there was no shoulder—just a drop down a ledge. My left knee and left foot took a beating from the jumps down to avoid oncoming cars.

At the bottom of this one-mile downhill, I saw a sign reading, "Mental Health Center Straight Ahead." I also saw that the road went straight up, which meant that the cars traveling downhill toward me would be coming faster. I felt about ready to check in at the Mental Health Center when I reached the top.

From the top of the hill, I saw nothing but mountains. Fort Payne lay in a narrow valley, so there was no way out except by crossing those mountains.

Fort Payne has a long history. The fort was built by order of General Winfield Scott and named after a Captain John Payne who was stationed here. It dates from 1848.

Some of the present town reflects this history. The town also lays claim to Sequoyah, an Indian genius who conceived and perfected (over a 12-year period) in its entirety an alphabet (84 letters).

Because of this alphabet, most of the Cherokee nation could read and write. The giant Sequoia trees and Sequoia National Park were named in his honor, though not staying true to the spelling of his name.

Going out of Fort Payne was as rough as coming into it—a long uphill pull. But I was rewarded with great views of the town nestled in the narrow valley.

Other than some of the worst road conditions I've experienced in weeks, there was really nothing unusual about the day. It simply moved us one day closer to the Atlantic.

There, come to think about it, is the big difference between normal life at home and life on this run. At home, the day is crowded with many chores—a number of which don't get done. Daily life at home is filled with shades of gray.

By contrast, here on the road we live in simple blacks and whites. All we have to accomplish is the daily mileage. If we log 26 miles on a day and don't wind up with an injury, it's a success.

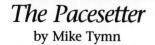

# E  S  S  A  Y

## *The Pacesetter*
by Mike Tymn

*(Mike is one of the leading authorities on running among the older age groups. He writes columns for* National Masters News, Running Times *and the* Honolulu Advertiser. *I have a special fondness for him because he's a fellow ex-Marine. — Paul Reese.)*

It wasn't too many years ago when vigorous physical activity was strictly within the domain of the young. From the world of sports, we had learned that humans were over the hill at 35 and washed up at 40.

Beyond the early 40s, we knew very little as to our capabilities in the areas of speed, strength, endurance and agility, as there had been no arena in which to test these attributes. Men were pretty much considered candidates for the rocking chair by 50 and were labeled "old geezers" by 60.

The running and fitness boom, kicked off by Dr. Kenneth Cooper and his 1968 book *Aerobics*, changed all that. The message preached by Dr. Cooper was one of lifetime fitness.

More and more middle-aged men and women took to the roads to "jog," as fitness running came to be called. But within a few years, some of these men—the more goal-oriented ones, perhaps—began looking for ways to test themselves and then to see how far they could push their limits. Thus masters competition, for men and women over 40, was born in the late 1960s.

Paul Reese took up running in the BC (Before Cooper) era. As a Marine Corps officer, he had come to appreciate the feeling that accompanies a high standard of physical fitness and to recognize the need for a program to maintain it for life.

Upon retiring from the Corps in 1963, he began running

to stay in shape. However, it wasn't until after Cooper and the advent of masters racing that Paul had an arena—one to motivate him to search for his limits. By that time, he was well into his 50s.

Paul quickly established himself as one of the three or four best in the world in his age-group. He set numerous American records at distances from five kilometers to 100 miles, and won many national championships.

At the age of 54, he ran a marathon in 2:39:28. For those not fully tuned to the running scene, that's an average of little more than six minutes a mile for 26.2 miles. It's a time that would have won the gold medal in seven Olympic Games and a pace that the average high school male cannot run for a single mile.

Paul continued setting records in older age groups. But he's more than a record-setter.

He was a pacesetter, a pioneer in the field of aging and athletic performance. He was one of the first men his age who pushed the limits of human performance far beyond what had been recognized as possible.

Paul served as an example and role model to many younger men and women, including myself. Although I had often read of his accomplishments over the years, the first time I watched him run was at the 1987 National Masters Championships in Eugene, Oregon.

He had turned 70 a few months before and was running 5000 meters on the track. I remember thinking, "What an elegant runner he is!" I admired the rhythm and vitality in his smooth stride.

It was then that I adopted Paul as one of my role models, one of my heroes. As I lag 20 years behind him, I have his example to guide me while I strive to grow old gracefully, vigorously and with dignity.

# *Overview of Georgia*

**August 6 to August 18, 1990 — 321.2 miles — 3104.3 total**

| Day | Overnight | Miles | Notes |
|-----|-----------|-------|-------|
| 108 | nr. Summerville | 26.4 | last 14.0 miles in Georgia |
| 109 | Calhoun | 26.4 | |
| 110 | Canton | 26.3 | |
| 111 | Alpharette | 26.4 | |
| 112 | near Russell | 26.6 | |
| 113 | near Rutledge | 26.5 | |
| 114 | Rutledge | 26.6 | temperature hit 102 degrees, met Frank Bacon |
| 115 | Crawfordsville | 26.8 | temperature 101 |
| 116 | Thompson | 26.7 | temperature 101 |
| 117 | near Wrens | 26.6 | temperature 100 |
| 118 | Waynesboro | 26.8 | |
| 119 | Sylvania | 26.6 | completed 3000 miles |

(first 14.9 miles in Georgia on Day 120)

## Chapter 11

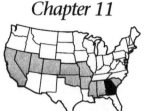

# Marching Through Georgia

Our next-to-last state would be no piece of cake. At about 320 miles, to be covered between August 6 and 18, it would be the longest crossing since Kansas.

I couldn't help envying George Billingsley. Reports had filtered back to me that he was approaching the Atlantic. At this rate, he would reach his finish line while I still faced another week on the road.

The highlight of Georgia would be a planned rendezvous with an old Marine Corps compadre of mine, Frank Bacon. His would be the first familiar face we'd seen in months.

**DAY 108.** As I stepped out of the motor home to begin running this morning, three thoughts jumped immediately to mind:

1. Traffic into Fort Payne at this early hour was excessively heavy. I hoped this wouldn't be the order of the day. (It wasn't.)

2. The skies suggested we were in for rain. Light rain is no problem, but a drenching thunderstorm like yesterday's washes away my enthusiasm. (No rain fell.)

3. Onward to Georgia today. That raised the morale flag quite a bit. (I'm now writing from our next-to-last state.)

By our calculations, we have 323 miles to get through Georgia. At the rate of 26.2 per day that translates to 12-1/2 days. Then comes a 90-mile victory lap through South Carolina.

One thing I'll say about the Alabama folks before leaving them behind: Judging from their waving and honking, they seem to be aware that we are doing what our RUNXUSA T-shirts say. That type of awareness did not prevail earlier as we crossed the South.

Well, in my body assessment this morning the good news was that I was still alive. The bad news was that I seemed to have muscle strains in the quads of both legs.

The spirit was willing; I felt aggressive. But the flesh was weak, because every time I tried to pick up the pace the quads rebelled.

This problem eased—only to be replaced by my old nemesis, knee pain. My left knee objected rather violently to a two-mile downhill drop. Downhill is an easy way to add miles but a hard way to preserve the body.

Usually, this knee will act up for a half-hour or so, then the pain will subside. Today, it persisted.

Then, sudden as a rifle shot, a pain hit the outside of my right knee, shooting down to my toes and paralyzing them for a second. I stumbled and almost fell, walked 20 steps and was back to normal. Figure that one.

My underlying thought at this stage of the game: Wouldn't it be a helluva note to get this far into a run across the country and have something happen that aborted it?

We must be nearing Jimmy Carter territory. Near the Alabama-Georgia border, we saw the first signs advertising boiled peanuts.

At the next pit stop beside a general store, guess who was sitting in the motor home munching boiled peanuts when I arrived. Elaine reported, "They taste somewhat like beans."

In the store, I saw something I've not seen for years—a punchout board that awards prizes for lucky numbers. Since the proprietor was kind enough to let me use his phone for a credit-card call, I bought a couple of $1 punches. No luck there.

But we got lucky on our routing. County Road 15 to the Georgia line turned out to be one of our best choices in a long while. I had the whole road to myself.

The first sight to catch my eye in Georgia was a cemetery with a large monument reading "Reese." A little spooky to see my name on a tombstone, especially as tired as I was.

After finishing in Summerville, we drove to James H. "Sloppy" Floyd State Park. It's named for a former Georgia state representative. The best feature of the park is the shower/ toilet facilities, all tile and spotlessly clean. Hey, Floyd, nothing sloppy about that!

Elaine and I agreed tonight about the biggest disappointment of the trip: the little recreational time we get after the running is done. By the time we locate an RV place, have our showers, have dinner, do this writing, and check the routing and camping possibilities for the next day, it's bedtime.

**DAY 109.** Heavy on my mind as I started this morning in the darkness at Summerville was, "How will that left knee behave today?" The pain had never been as intense as it was yesterday, nor had it persisted for so long.

Concerned about what today would bring, I tried a different pair of inserts—the soft orthopedic Spencos. Two miles down, and the knee wasn't balking even though the arthritic foot was touchy. Hell, I could run through that, but a wounded knee would be debilitating.

At five miles, still no distress signals from the knee. The morale flag was fluttering merrily in the breeze.

And so it went all day. The knee that had troubled me for the last 20 miles yesterday bothered me not at all today. The soft Spencos must have worked.

Sometimes, while trying to hold myself together, I feel like a pilot going over a checklist: (1) Is the sacroiliac belt fastened tightly? (2) Need any Aspercreme? (3) How about suntan lotion? (4) Blistex—got some on? Remember how chapped and cut those lips were in Nevada and Utah? (5) Water bottle filled? (6) Injury assessment? (7) Carrying some repellent for mosquitoes and chiggers?

In Summerville this morning, I saw my first runner in weeks. He was on his morning outing, and we had a brief talk. I didn't mention running across the USA.

One of the most distressing sights on this run has been the hundreds of animals killed on the highways. Today, I saw two dead dogs, then in the last mile I passed a dead cat.

Most animals killed on the highway look anguished. But this cat looked blissfully serene, almost as if to say, "Welcome, Death."

After viewing this carnage, I'm noting with relief that about 50 percent of the drivers were moving over for me today. That was up from the 10 percent of yesterday.

At the last pit stop, I told Elaine, "I can't understand why I'm so fast today." She looked at my watch, then kindly reminded me, "You forgot to move it ahead from Central to Eastern time."

We're spending the night at a KOA campground. Sterile camping compared to the Alabama and Georgia state parks, and almost twice as costly.

But that is the consistency of KOA. You can always expect it to be overpriced.

**DAY 110.** On the phone last night, daughter Susan told us, "All arrangements are made for your four-night cruise. Royal Caribbean to the Bahamas."

Now it's imperative that we finish on time to catch that cruise ship. Egad, what a mess if there's a delay!

Being on the western edge of a new time zone made our start unusually dark at 5:50 this morning. Instead of veering away from me, many of the drivers edged toward me—probably to get a better look at this creature in the darkness.

The morning flow of traffic east toward Interstate 75 was fast and furious. Commuters hurried to work at the big manufacturing companies along the I-75 corridor.

This hectic stretch of road again verified my observation from across the country that truck drivers come in two types. Either they're very courteous, swinging wide to give me running room, or they're sadistic, trying to scare me by not giving an inch.

My first mistake of the day came when I tried to reach a road construction site before work started there. Moving too fast before I was warmed up, my left knee complained, "Hey, wait a minute, boy!"

After smooth sailing yesterday, it was a bit discouraging to start off today with the knee a bit flaky. But I did beat the construction workers.

My reward was a run on a new, unopened road. I owned this road and ran my best mile of the day on it.

The left knee must have decided I wouldn't put up with any of its foolishness. It settled into half-hearted whimpering.

By 20 miles, both knees were complaining about how tired they were. I replied, "Shut up! I'm tired, too."

Old legs are tiring in wornout shoes. I'm hoping to receive new ones at our mail pickup in Lawrenceville, Georgia. But if I don't and have to finish in these old shoes, you can call me "Mr. Wobbles."

This was a day for the birds. At a pit stop, Elaine parked beside a pond that was home to geese and ganders.

To their delight, she fed them cornmeal muffins. Leaving the pit stop, I heard them honking for more handouts.

Poultry farming is big in this area. I saw several farms with hundreds of chickens, all huddled together.

Some of the poultry sheds sit close to the road. Believe me, they're odiferous.

These sheds are 100 or more yards long with tin roofs, doors at each end and screened sides. Each shed has a couple of grain bins that pump feed to the birds inside.

I stopped to talk with one poultry farmer. He said, "One shed can house as many as 17,000 chickens."

We noticed that many homes in this area carry wreaths on the front door. Elaine and I have seen so many of these in the South that we've concluded they are welcome wreaths and not left over from Christmas.

Elaine didn't have a restful day on the road. At one point, she encountered a sign reading "Tunnel ahead, 9'6" high."

She fretted about the motor home passing under that ceiling. But it went through with inches to spare, and I found her parked on the other side with a relieved and proud smile on her face.

Later, an oil truck tailgated her so closely that she had a risky time making a left turn without getting hit. Too bad there's not a way to shake up some of these truck drivers as much as they unsettle us.

The running day ended with three miles in a thunderstorm and rain. With no RV parks in the area, we drove to Canton and are overnighting at a Day's Inn. We'll go to bed thinking, "Only 14 days left."

**DAY 111.** Foggy and very dark out here this morning as I give a running account of my day to the tape recorder. Always wonder as I go down the road like this, highway forest growth on both sides of the road, how many animal eyes are looking at me and how many creatures are thinking, "What's this?"

I start off with so much anxiety about the darkness and safety that I failed to notice until this moment. I'm running without any signs of my usual latent injuries.

The world's awakening. I hear the roosters as I pass a poultry ranch and its sheds—which, incidentally, are kept lighted all night.

In Waleska, I go by Rinehart College which was founded in 1883. I get the impression that it stresses academics.

I doubt if it even has a football team. I know that it's not on Notre Dame's schedule. About the only distraction in this hamlet for students is a convenience store.

Going through this town, I pass a home with five unlocked bicycles sitting on the front porch. Can't imagine that in any big USA city today. The bikes would disappear instantly.

Well, here's a political development I was not abreast of. "Re-elect Lester Maddox Governor in 1990," reads a poster.

Let me tell you, they have mosquitoes here in Georgia. Hungry mosquitoes. This moment, they're feasting on my California blood.

I go by Cherokee High School and experience a moment of excitement. At first glance, I think the athletic stadium is called "Tammy Baker Field." Then I see it's named for a TOMMY Baker.

Even though school has not opened yet, the majorettes are out practicing. I can see they're big on football here with their night lights and stadium that must seat at least 8000.

Now as we go into Canton, the highway is lined with middle-class and upper-middle-class homes. This is not a country backroad anymore but a heavily traveled commute route. I suppose that much of this fury results from the area being within commuting distance of Atlanta.

Stepping up to enter the motor home at the 15-mile pit stop, I get my first hamstring pull in 109 days of running. I've had hints of it coming for over a month. Anytime I stretch out in bed at night, the hamstring will tie up and I'll have to massage out the knot.

A happy thought crosses my mind as I again jump out to the weeds. Just how many times can I do this without stepping on a snake? If I do, he'd better be careful because I'm in a mood to bite him back.

Well, this is a win-some/lose-some day. We win on the weather with the overcast lasting until noon. When the sun does come out, the weather is not overly hot.

But we lose on traffic, heavy as it is all day. The last two miles today are the most aggravating I've run in weeks.

After we finish this transcon run, it will be a long time—if ever—before I get out on a highway and run facing a stream of fast traffic. One piece of advice I'd give to anyone contemplating a transcon run: There is considerable inherent danger.

After hunting unsuccessfully for an RV park, Elaine and I locate only one motel—the Marriott Residence. The nightly rate, the clerk tells us, is $120.

"Uh, no thanks," Elaine says. "It's not the price. We're just not dressed properly in our T-shirts and running shorts."

So we're spending the night in a quiet corner of a shopping plaza. We're quite comfortable here. And, yeah, $120 richer.

**DAY 112.** The advice of my Marine Corps friend Frank Bacon now rings in my ears. "If you get anywhere near Atlanta, the traffic will snow you under," he had warned. Too true today!

The commute traffic this morning was horrendous. I witnessed in hundreds of cars the stress, the cigarette smoking, the coffee drinking, the frenzy, the grimness of these people hurrying to work.

Out here in suburbia, the forestry is eye-catching. But making this commute daily would be an ulcer producer.

By moving over just one foot, which they easily could have done, these drivers would have allowed me to run on the road. But none were inclined to do that.

They displayed the discourteous big-city mentality. In the USA, the jungles are in the cities, not in the rural areas.

The commute traffic was heavily sprinkled with BMWs and Mercedes. Seeing them I thought, "If I'm going to get hit, let it be by one of these rich dudes or dames."

The same thought occurred to me as I saw a sign at an estate reading, "Patrol dogs." If I'm going to get bitten, that's the kind of a dog I want to do it, and then I want a good liability attorney on my side.

I can't remember going by so many luxurious homes—all with expansive acreage, gates, alarms, all the trimmings—as I saw in the affluent Atlanta suburb of Alpharette. At one home, the grounds were so extensive that at first glance I thought it was a golf course.

A little farther down the highway, I passed a place called "Recreation World, Family Entertainment Center." It advertised a 54-hole miniature golf course, its four waterfalls visible from the road. Left me wondering: Just how long does it take to play 54 holes?

Golf is but one of the center's many attractions. Something this big has to be supported by the natives of Atlanta.

Next, I came to the River Exchange, a huge shopping mall. Whatever happened to the back roads and boondocks?

And with all the affluence in these parts, why are the roads so damnably narrow? Some of the trucks actually overhang the road.

To be on the roads I've traveled the past few days, a runner is not very smart. For a bicyclist to use them would be insane. Maybe that's why I've seen neither.

If General Sherman had had as much trouble marching through Georgia as I've had running through this state the past few days, the Civil War would still be going on.

The battle cry today was, "On to Lawrenceville and our Georgia mail call." Contemplating the mail pickup made me realize that in our planning Elaine and I made a major mistake.

Before starting, we should have designated one city in each state as our mail-pickup point and then given family and friends that list of cities. We've done this by phone for our family with the last three states and it has worked well, but we've fallen badly out of touch with our friends.

At least one thing worked out today as planned. We finished directly in front of the Lawrenceville Post Office and went inside to collect our prizes.

**DAY 113.** I was running along wearily on a divided highway when three guys in a pickup approached. Trying to scare me, they veered off toward me and into the weeds.

As they got close, one of them banged the metal door of the pickup. I jumped farther into the weeds to escape them.

All this aroused my Marine Corps fighting blood. I gave them the European obscene gesture after they'd gone by.

That, I thought, was the end of it. But about three minutes later, I saw the same pickup approaching me on the other side of the median.

It crossed the median strip and headed toward me again. "Uh oh, here comes trouble," I thought.

To avoid it—after all, there were three of them and my Marine Corps fighting blood is no longer youthful—I ran across the grass median and started moving with traffic. The pickup stopped, and one of the guys got out and yelled, "You gave me the finger!"

Trying to placate him, I shouted back, "Sorry about the gesture, but you scared the hell out of me." Then I realized that the guy bordered on being drunk.

He surprised me by saying, "If I had seen how old you are, I wouldn't have done that." I liked the non-threatening tone of that.

"You know," I said, "you could have killed me. I might have spooked, jumped the wrong way and crashed into your truck."

"Oh, hell," he answered, "we were just fooling around. Sorry."

We talked a bit, and finally he said, "Okay, let's shake hands and be friends."

I met him midway in the median and we shook hands. Next, he insisted on hugging me and again told me how sorry he was.

I now realized this guy was blotto. He wanted to hug me a couple more times, and I worried that he might want to kiss.

Finally, I yelled to the other two guys in the truck, "You'd better get him out of here, or people will be talking about us."

As he left, I was able to smile over this experience that enlivened my day. It also reminded me to restrain myself in the future.

After all, he could have come back with a shotgun or a .38. Visions of "Easy Rider" passed through my mind.

Later today, three old ladies in a Cadillac pulled up alongside me. The driver, taking a cigarette out of her mouth, asked, "How old are you?"

I said, "You guess." But she was polite and didn't, so I told her.

"You're in great shape for your age," she said. "How far have you run?"

I told her I'd come from California and was headed for the Atlantic Ocean.

"Oh, you're pulling my leg," she replied.

"No, it's true," I said, then told her about Elaine who was ahead of me. Suddenly, the women in the Cadillac seemed to lose interest and drove off.

Surprisingly, they returned a short while later and said they'd called the local newspaper, but no one answered the phone. They now wanted to interview me themselves.

I answered a few questions, then told them, "I have to start running because Elaine will get nervous if I don't show on time."

One of the ladies said diplomatically, "We're honored to have you run through our town." A second one added, not diplomatically, "Especially at your age!"

Elaine told me at the next pit stop that they had tracked her down for an interview. Elaine reported that when they asked my age it was to satisfy a bet among them.

One of them had said, "He'll never see 70 again." That didn't help my self-image.

**DAY 114.** The new shoes I broke in yesterday proved to be a disappointment. I'd expected them to work magic but discovered they were a half-size too small. My feet have expanded by one full shoe size since California.

My only course of action was to perform surgery on these brand-new shoes. I cut out the toebox to make my growing feet comfortable.

One problem with these shoes with the toebox cut out is that pieces of dirt and gravel fly into the open toebox and cut into my feet. Stiff as I am these days, it's difficult to stop on the highway, remove the shoe and extract the irritant. I'd give ransom money for a pair of shoes that fit.

Going along today, I found myself disassociating again to take my mind off the battle being waged to keep running. I reviewed my overriding impressions of the states we've passed through.

California: the excitement of starting at Jenner, the sendoff by friends who ran the Slice 100-K race with us, the snow at Carson Pass.

Nevada: the beautiful sunrises and sunsets of the desert, the surprise of so many mountains over 6000-feet elevation.

Utah: the caring people, the spectacular colors in the mountains.

Colorado: the majestic peaks, the many clear streams, the white water of the Arkansas River.

Kansas: the wheat fields and harvesting, the friendly people.

Oklahoma: the need for improvement on all counts.

Missouri: the surprising beauty of the Ozarks, more friendly people.

Arkansas: more of the Ozark mountains and their enchantment.

Mississippi: the poverty of some of its people, the elation of running over the Mississippi River.

Alabama: the cotton and soybean fields.

Georgia: the miserable road and traffic conditions near Atlanta, the thick forestation.

Doing a bit more meditating as I moved along, I pinpointed the remaining milestones. The first will be reaching the 3000-mile mark in a couple of days, the next when we enter South Carolina and the final one when we splash into the Atlantic Ocean.

But where would that splashdown come? Elaine and I agreed

today that a final decision is long overdue.

Indecisiveness is getting to us. And our family, friends and Marine compadres in Georgia want to know where we will finish. Decision time.

We've discarded our original choice of Savannah, Georgia, as impractical. But we haven't yet chosen among several possible alternative finish lines.

Charleston, South Carolina, is one. I have a good friend there, and General Mark Clark once had offered me a job at the Citadel. Charleston is rich in history, but as we studied Charleston the approaches looked difficult.

Our research also revealed that Beaufort, South Carolina, is closer and there I have a genuine connection: Finish at the Marine Corps Air Station at Beaufort.

But during the past week or so as the Persian Gulf situation has developed, I've begun to have doubts about MCAS, Beaufort. This station has more important matters to deal with than an ancient, retired Marine Corps officer finishing his run across the USA there.

That in mind, Elaine and I studied the maps for landing sites near Beaufort. Hilton Head Island caught our eye.

Charleston is out. Beaufort is a gamble. Hilton Head is a sure thing.

What's more, Elaine and I will want some immediate rest and recreation after we finish. The resort area of Hilton Head is an easy winner.

Onward, Christian soldier, to Hilton Head Island! There, by the grace of God, we'll splash down 10 days from now.

**DAY 115.** We started in front of the Sugar Creek Baptist Church—founded in 1833. This was a fitting beginning, because God was smiling on this enterprise today.

A quarter of a mile later, a farmer seeing me run by Elaine's headlights on this dark and foggy morning, stopped to ask if we needed help. Such offers have come rarely in Georgia.

A short while later, after Elaine had driven ahead, I could see the outlines of a lake. A sign informed me that two miles from this spot Fort Matthews was built in 1793. That's getting to the roots of our history.

The traffic was so light that I could enjoy the beauty of this area. Going down the road at first light, all by myself, I was swayed by the beauty of the scene and heard myself spontaneously saying, "God, You made a beautiful world! Too bad people keep messing it up."

A day that started this perfectly just had to contain the happiest event in a long time. Elaine and I were enjoying a snack at a pit stop when a car pulled up nearby.

We saw two men walking toward us. It took me a moment to see that they weren't more strangers stopping to chat or to ask if we were okay.

One was Frank Bacon, a Marine Corps buddy of mine. Frank, a retired colonel, lives nearby in Milledgeville, Georgia.

He and his brother Paul had come out to welcome us to their state. When we'd corresponded before the run started, Frank had said, "I'll meet you on the road." Sure enough, here he was.

Frank and I were in the same Marine Corps officers' class, the 7th ROC, and we were both commissioned second lieutenants in January 1942. Frank's whole purpose in driving out here was to visit with us.

We talked for a pleasant hour. Frank arranged for us to meet with him and his wife Margie for dinner tomorrow night.

As Frank was about to leave, I asked, "Why don't you run a few miles with me?" He had been on the University of Georgia cross-country team in his youth but told me, "My knees don't tolerate running these days."

As Frank drove off, Elaine and I felt our spirits elevated by his visit. I, like all the other survivors of the 7th ROC, know this caring to be typical of Frank.

As president of our association, he has worked diligently over the years to plan the annual reunions which bring joy to all of us. It's quite emotional to visit classmates you've known since 1942—men who, like you, speak the language of World War II, the Marine Corps dialect.

Frank's visit and the anticipation of another to come carried me through this day of oppressively humid heat. At times, I felt fuzzy, dizzy, even on the verge of passing out.

But the human body, I've learned through years of running, is a remarkable piece of machinery—capable of much more than the guy who holds the warranty on it generally realizes.

**DAY 116.** My mind drifts back to mulling the decision of where to finish our run—Beaufort or Hilton Head Island—and how that distraction eased the running and passed the time a couple of days ago. Why not try the same thing today? What I'll do is dwell on some conclusions about running across the

USA—or better, advice to people thinking of making such a run.

1. It's useless to undertake it unless you design it for enjoyment. If your only desire is to run across the country as fast as possible, to see nothing in particular, to take the shortest route, maybe you should consider going by airplane.

2. It's imperative that you and your pit-crew person are 100-percent compatible. You're a team. Any runner who thinks he can make it without good pit-crewing is foolhardy.

3. On a run across the USA, there is no free lunch. You'll face heat, cold, cars, insects and other adversaries. Be prepared to handle the unexpected.

4. Your biggest problem will be finding running space. Avoid big cities and their environs, of course, but even the back roads can be treacherous.

5. Oh yeah, it wouldn't be a bad idea to take out a life insurance policy since there is so much inherent danger.

6. It's a good idea to keep a log of some sort. As the days go on, it's hard to remember what happened where and when.

7. Don't think in terms of 3000 miles. Approach the days one at a time. Actually, as you go along you'll most likely find yourself thinking of making it from one pit stop to the next.

The list could go on. But that number 3000 triggered another thought. This was an epochal day for us because we hit 3000 miles, meaning we have only 190 or so to go.

That's an elevating thought. But as I've said many times before, it's not in the bag until we run into the Atlantic.

I remind myself to be careful with only eight or nine days left. Don't get too eager and run myself into an injury.

Speaking of being prepared for the unexpected: We had planned to finish near Warrenton, check into a motel there and then meet Frank and Margie Bacon for dinner.

We found no motel and had to drive 13 miles to Thompson to locate one. After showering and dressing, we returned to Warrenton for dinner.

The Bacons met us at the restaurant, said it had slipped since they last ate there and suggested that we drive to another— yes, back in Thompson, two blocks from our motel. That's how it goes when you're running across the USA.

But our dinner with Frank and Margie more than made up for the confusion. They told us that some Marine Corps friends were planning a dinner for us in Savannah on August 25 and a luncheon the next day at the Skidaway Island Country Club.

After a couple of months without seeing anyone we knew, our social calendar is picking up!

Elaine and I returned to our motel tonight harboring a warm feeling for the finishing touches these festivities will add to our run. We were thinking we'd be on a high when we finished and that it would be normal for a letdown to follow. But now, anticipating the get-togethers with good friends, we see little chance of that happening.

**DAY 117.** During our conversation, Frank reported great news. A Savannah TV station had shown George Billingsley running into the Atlantic at Tybee Island to finish his trek across the USA.

"He looked wildly jubilant," said Frank. And well he should have, I thought.

He'd covered 3028 miles. Subtracting the first ceremonial day he ran with me, George had averaged 26.33 miles for 115 days. By taking the direct route after parting company with us, he was able to save 164 miles.

To me, the distinctive feature of George's run was the courage he displayed. From the time he reached Nevada until he finished at South Carolina, he was plagued with injuries—either a knee or shin splints—that forced him to walk many hours each day.

I found myself thinking a lot about Frank Bacon today. Frank deserves tremendous credit for welding together all the survivors of our 7th Marine Corps Reserve Officers Class (ROC). It's quite a kaleidoscope of characters.

After we became second lieutenants in 1942, we received our assignments. Those who lived west of the Mississippi were sent to Camp Elliott or Camp Pendleton in California, and all from east of the Mississippi were sent to Camp LeJeune, North Carolina. Those who went east were in the units that made the initial landing at Guadalcanal the following August, so very early we lost classmates there. We lost others at each of the island campaigns.

After the war, some of these men stayed in the Corps, some did not. Almost all those in civilian life seem to have done well—presidents and vice-presidents of companies, attorneys, MDs, businessmen.

Frank has kept this group in touch by publishing a newsletter over the years, and during the past decade we've held an annual reunion. Because of our vintage now, with different classmates dying each year, I'm moved to sometimes wonder, "Why he and not me?" Just as in war.

We're now committed to finishing on August 22. We promised Frank Bacon and Joe Hall, who are handling publicity for our finish at Hilton Head Island, that we would run into the Atlantic at 10 a.m.

Elaine announced this morning, "I've done some calculating. After today, we have five more 26-mile days, then a 19 and just five miles on the final day."

Elaine's news is encouraging. But we do feel a little pressure over having to arrive at Hilton Head at a specific date and hour.

As the days wind down, I reflect more and more on what RUNXUSA has meant to me. I think how fortunate I am to be able to experience this run, especially at my age—fortunate to be able to handle it physically and financially, fortunate to have the time to do it and blessed to have Elaine's help.

She has done countless things to ease the run for me. I smile while thinking of the root beer float that waits for me at the end of each day's run and which I savor as we drive towards an RV park for the night.

Never before has anyone been beside me over so long a period of time with us both zeroed in on accomplishing the same goal. Our togetherness and harmony brings me more pleasure than anything on this trip.

But I'll be glad to get it over. I'm tired. I've got sleep to catch up on.

Elaine says, "If after we finish you mention getting up early, I'll kill you." By that standard, I should live a long time.

**DAY 118.** I've been trying to think of some analogy to describe how tired I am these days and have come up with this one. I feel like a guy who, when he started in the Pacific, felt like he had the strength and size of Arnold Schwarzenegger. When he finishes in the Atlantic, he'll feel like he has the strength and size of George Burns.

Reflecting some more today on RUNXUSA, I realize that we've been damn lucky. We've kept our health, had no accidents, and overall the weather has been kind enough to bring us no severe storms.

Even the dogs have cooperated. I calculate that by now a thousand dogs must have barked at me. Remarkably, not one has attacked. Bless the magic word, "Stay!"

Thinking back on a conversation we had last night, I

mentioned Bruce Tulloh's book, *Four Million Footsteps*. He was a world-class runner who ran across the country in a remarkable 65 days back in 1969.

Talking about Tulloh's run made me curious about how many footsteps I would take across the USA while running a distance about 300 miles longer than his and with a much shorter stride. I calculated it at somewhere around ten million steps.

Several people have asked me, "How are you able to do 26 miles day after day?" I'm not sure whether they're thinking about the distance or my age, but I have yet to give a serious answer to that question. I usually dismiss it with a joking remark like, "One step at a time."

The serious answer, I guess, has something to do with mindset—the desire, dedication, determination to just do it, believing I can, hanging in there each day, giving no thought to quitting until I do it.

From that, I made an abrupt transition to thinking about the primitive nature of our trek by foot across the continent as the Indians and pioneers did. It doesn't get much more basic than that.

On second thought, that might be blasphemy to them. They didn't have the luxury of a motor home for pit stops and evenings.

A young black guy drove past me today, stopped, stuck his head out the car window and took a long look at me. His expression said with no words being needed, "I can't believe this."

"Fellow, I'm with you," I thought. There are times when Elaine and I can hardly believe this run ourselves.

So much has stacked up that I can't remember day-to-day events and places. Thank God I've kept this log to resurrect all that.

Oh sure, some unusual events like crossing Monarch Pass or the Mississippi River, and some unusual places like Austin, Nevada, or Royal Gorge, Colorado, are distinct memories. But at this point, so much time and distance have passed that I need the log to unravel what happened when and where. For sure, there would be no other way that Elaine or I could convey to family and friends the magnitude of what we've been through.

Nor do we expect people to understand even after they read this log. That's sort of like trying to get a man to understand what it's like to go through childbirth, or like getting a person who has never heard a shot fired in anger to understand combat.

**DAY 119.** We feasted last night for bargain-basement prices at a lakeside restaurant. For $4.49 each, Elaine and I had chicken with dumplings, potatoes, two different vegetables, coconut cake, ice cream, soup and a trip to the salad bar—not in that order, I must mention.

Elaine felt proud of herself this morning, and justifiably so. She'd finished a major sewing project which consisted of making a blue, floral-print, cotton dress and a purse to match.

She was inspired to undertake this project because she needs clothes to wear on the cruise we hadn't anticipated taking when we left home. She modeled for me last night, and I must say her creations are professional.

In the course of a pit stop conversation today, I asked Elaine, "What has been the toughest thing on the whole trip for you?" You know what mine was: finding running space on the road.

Without hesitation, Elaine replied, "The heat." That surprised me. I had expected her to say, "Finding a place to park the motor home for pit stops."

As for heat, no doubt we made a major mistake in our planning by not getting a motor home with a generator to keep it cool while Elaine was parked and waiting.

Running along today, I kept seeing a crop that I couldn't identify. Neither could Elaine.

At the next pit stop, we met a 12-year-old boy who told us the crop was peas. Elaine had a long conversation with this boy named Nicky and learned that the zenith of his life is visiting the Dairy Queen in Waynesboro.

Nicky's rotund shape testified to the fact that he didn't go there just to talk. He also told us about "a great place" in Girard to get a Coke and mentioned being a frequent visitor there, too.

Today's report from the animal kingdom, living and otherwise: A sow pig with her brood of nine piglets crossed the road and headed up the highway towards us at a pit stop. Elaine swore they were wild.

We captured the pigs on the camcorder just before they charged into the woods. I was glad to see them get off the highway before they were baconized.

When I reached the next pit stop, Elaine was parked about

100 yards from where a doe had been killed by a car. Thirty to 40 vultures were feasting on the carcass, and others were perched in a nearby tree that was naked of foliage. A macabre scene.

Much on our minds today is that we are edging toward South Carolina, the last of our 12 states. We didn't quite make it today, falling about six miles short.

But that will be The Happening tomorrow. We'll soon be able to smell the Atlantic.

After today's run, Elaine and I drove into South Carolina to scout the bridge over the Savannah River and to pick up tourist information at that state's Welcome Center.

Returning to Georgia, we stopped at its Welcome Center to collect data on Savannah, where we will be spending a couple of days and nights socializing after leaving Hilton Head.

From the Georgia Welcome Center, it was a 16-mile drive to Sylvania—our closest connection to an RV park. We go to bed tonight with sweet dreams of South Carolina.

# E S S A Y

## *The Runnerup*
### by George Billingsley

*(No higher compliment can I give George than to say he would have made a damned good Marine. He was "wounded" early in his campaign to get from the Pacific to the Atlantic— first running through a case of shin splints, then encountering problems with a knee that had undergone surgery twice. Yet he never took his eyes off the target. If George had gone 2000 miles before incurring an injury, his resolve to finish would have been understandable. But the injuries descended on him before he'd completed 10 percent of the journey. Under these circumstances, most of us would have surrendered. But that is not the nature of George Billingsley. Like a Marine, he was going forward until the mission was accomplished. — Paul Reese.)*

**August 15:** Here's the letter I promised 65 days ago in Colorado when we took different routes and I said I'd get in touch when I finished. I was disappointed that you didn't come with me on a more direct route. Nonetheless, I have many fond memories of our more than 1300 miles together.

Without your company, I began to think increasingly less like a butterfly flitting from flower to flower and more like a hornet headed for a bare ass. For business and personal reasons, Georgia wanted to get home as soon as possible, and so did I.

We spent some evenings studying the maps for the best route. We chose the straightest and best running course possible without compromising our guidelines:

1. To keep the route continuous and not skip a single footstep.
2. To average a marathon a day.
3. To take no days off.

I walked and ran whenever possible on the edge of Interstate freeways. Georgia and I found this was the least offensive to motorists, and was by far the safest for both foot traffic and parking our Minnie Winnie motor home.

Unfortunately, there wasn't a continuous route of Interstates leading to our finish at Tybee Island, Georgia. Our route to the Atlantic Ocean beach contained hundreds of miles of secondary roads where there is no shoulder for running or parking. By comparison, running on the shoulder of an Interstate was blissful.

My right knee troubled me for much of the journey. The pain was never enough to shut me down, but it did limit my running.

I had to walk a lot of the time (very embarrassing for a hard-core ultramarathoner). I told myself that getting the distance was all that mattered, but I didn't really believe it.

Interestingly, however, it seemed that the adversities stimulated me and intensified my resolve to finish. I knew that nothing, short of getting squashed by a truck, would keep me from eventually running into the Atlantic.

Throughout the trip, we coddled and respected the Minnie Winnie. We knew she was getting on in years, so every morning since Day One, I opened the hood, kissed her radiator and told her how sweet she was.

But in spite of my love and kindness, one day she sprung a leak in the radiator that got all those loving smooches. Getting Minnie fixed cost me three low-mileage days—one 19.4, one 14.8 and a 9.4. This brought the daily average down from 26.5 to 26.0 and made me mighty nervous.

We started the trip with three cats. Georgia would not leave home without them, so they came along. They made good traveling companions and kept Georgia company while I was out slogging down the road. To round out our family, we picked up a starving kitten from a recently disked wheat field in Kansas.

The last part of the journey was heavenly. Everything was, "Tybee Island, here we come!"

With Georgia at the helm, Minnie purring like Air Force One, the knee getting no worse, the body parts and cats singing harmony, we turtled our way forward.

We had finally captured the rhythm of the trip. By the time we hit the border of Georgia, with a mere 320 miles to go, I began to smell the salt air and hear the ladies, clad in their scant bikinis, chanting in unison, "Go, George, Go!"

My feet finally splashing into the Atlantic ranks as one of those events a guy will replay in his mind forever. It was made even sweeter because, in my case, there were times when our goal to cross the USA on foot seemed like the impossible dream.

My difficulties helped make my splash an emotional crescendo. When I regained my composure, my first reaction was to wade out of the ocean and give Georgia a hug and a kiss. She made it all possible.

Following that, our son Mike (he's studying to be an Episcopalian priest) led our East Coast family in a "Thank God we made it" ceremony. The people on the beach, the Tybee Island officials, police escort and TV crews joined in the celebration. I appreciated the fuss they made over our accomplishment.

I know that your victorious day is close at hand and that you are in for a natural high beyond description. It would have been even better for me if we could have charged into the ocean together.

As it is, I wish I could be there to cheer your finish. But that is not to be. Georgia has the throttle to the floor. With the bit in her teeth, she is headed for home with her four cats and skinny husband.

So here we are today, just after finishing, back-tracking the same course to Tybee Island beach that I covered on foot. Miles that took me days to eke out are flashing by in reverse order. It reminds me of fast-forward on the VCR.

I'm beginning to appreciate how much greater the experience of crossing the country on foot is than seeing things flash by at 60 miles per hour. Since the days of the pioneers, only a few of us have had such a close look at our magnificent country.

# Overview of South Carolina

**August 18 to 22, 1990 — 87.5 miles — 3192.6 total**

| Day | Overnight | Miles | Notes |
|-----|-----------|-------|-------|
| 120 | Estill | 26.7 | last 11.8 miles in S. Carolina |
| 121 | Point South | 26.6 | |
| 122 | Hilton Head Is. | 26.4 | ran last 26-mile day |
| 123 | Hilton Head Is. | 18.3 | RUNXUSA four months old |
| 124 | Hilton Head Is. | 5.2 | finished RUNXUSA at Atlantic |

*Chapter 12*

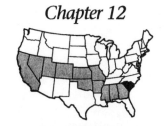

# Splashdown
# in South Carolina

So it had come down to this as we entered South Carolina:
Eleven states behind us, one to go.
Beyond 3100 miles, less than 100 to go.
One hundred and eighteen straight days averaging 26 miles,
three to go starting August 18 before the distances would tail
off for the long-anticipated finish on August 22.


**DAY 120.** Uppermost in our minds this foggy morning
was our crossing into South Carolina, our 12th and final state.
Its border was smack in the middle of the Savannah River.

We'd reconnoitered the bridge yesterday and found that
crossing it wouldn't be as difficult as anticipated. It's stimulating
now to count on the fingers of one hand the number of days
we have left.

Running toward the river, I was feeling the muscle strain
and tiredness that has dogged me the past week. Prior to that,
I'd been blessedly free of muscular problems.

Many pickups towed boats along the highway this Saturday
morning. Fishermen were heading for their favorite spots on
the Savannah River, I'd guess.

On the west edge of the bridge over the river, I stopped to
read a sign saying that in 1765 Robert Dunne began operating
a ferry here. This was a gateway to the west for the settlers
from the Carolinas and Virginia.

There was a guard rail all across the bridge, and along its
base a ledge about a foot wide and raised a foot above the
highway. These gave me safe passage and even allowed me to
stop midway to admire the view of the 300-yard-wide river
with thick tree growth on each side.

As always, we leave a state with a feeling of accomplishment, and we enter a state with a feeling of anticipation. Never has this been more true than today.

Shortly after setting foot in South Carolina, I heard shooting a short distance from the road. This set me to worrying that some damn fool could fire in my direction.

Parked at the pit stop Elaine talked to hunters who informed her that deer season opened today. Eek!

Later, my fears grew when some hunters stopped to ask me for directions to a hunting club. I thought, "If they're out here with guns and know nothing about the area, how do they know they're not shooting toward the highway?"

My stress level climbed even higher when I saw a sign reading, "Caution. High-powered rifles being used on Gray Plantation." What's that mean—we're supposed to stay off the road?

I passed by the South Carolina Welcome Center we'd visited yesterday. On our recon trip here, we'd collected information about Hilton Head Island.

It mainly told us that most of the beaches there are private. But no problem. We'd already decided to finish at Folly Field Beach, one of only two that's open to the public.

To pass the miles, I started thinking about running into Hilton Head Island. How difficult will it be to cross the bridge to the island? What road or traffic problems will I have getting from the bridge to Folly Field Beach?

As I thought about the potential for trouble in the final miles, I decided we would be smart to scout out the area the day before we finished there.

This practical thought led to a fanciful one: We will have close to 3200 miles when we finish. How much farther could I go?

Physically, I could go on, but psychologically I would weaken. I'd lose the will to continue quicker than I'd lose the physical ability.

We bought groceries tonight at a market where 90 percent of the shoppers were black. A middle-aged black man surprised me by asking, "Didn't I see you running on the road today?"

This cleared the way for a pleasant conversation. No day on the road is complete without one.

**DAY 121.** Thick fog as we started this morning. On the scene were hunters, and one stopped to ask if he could help us.

These hunters on the road give me cause for reflection. As a high school freshman, I spent part of my summer at my uncle Pros's ranch, assisting him with deer hunters.

My job was to guide the hunters to their stands. Then, working with his dogs, Uncle Pros would try to flush the deer towards the hunters.

How the years—and in my case, the experience of being shot at in war—do change us. Now my sympathies go to the deer. I wouldn't think of shooting one.

My obsession for these many miles has been with maintaining my own health. But now I'm concerned for Elaine.

Yesterday, she wrenched her back. This morning, she has a slight fever, serious enough to be irritating but not debilitating.

Police officers sure do dress informally around here. Parked for a pit stop this morning, Elaine had one stop to ask if she was in trouble. He was dressed in an orange T-shirt and shorts.

Later, one asked me if I needed help. He wore Levis, a T-shirt and a ball cap that said, "Dixie. God's country."

Whenever I go by a home on these back roads of the South and see somebody there, I always wave. Never has anybody failed to wave back.

If only the dogs were this friendly! Today, I came closest to being attacked during the entire trip.

Three dogs came out from under the porch of a shack and charged me. I yelled, "Stay!" but for once this trick didn't work. They kept advancing slowly, menacingly.

I reached down as if to pick up a weapon, and that fake halted the dogs momentarily. Then I found a stick and waved it threateningly, at the same time letting out a war whoop.

The dogs backed off. This was my clue to mount an offensive.

I moved toward them, waving the stick and letting out blood-curdling yells. Oh, blessed sight! They turned and retreated.

We're overnighting at a KOA campground. Overpriced, as always, but we're thankful it's available.

Speaking of money, Elaine took an accounting today. She reports, "Our daily expenses have averaged $40.49 which includes gas, food, lodging and incidentals."

Elaine and I talked this evening about how our daily routine has evolved in a most surprising way. Before leaving home, we'd planned on starting each day's run at about seven o'clock.

At the time, I thought that was really early. Yet after two weeks on the road, we found ourselves rolling out of bed between 4:00 and 4:30, and running within an hour by Elaine's headlights or my flashlight.

The modus operandi is that I run three miles, to where Elaine is parked for a pit stop. I eat and drink what she has prepared, and we visit. Then I shove off for another three miles.

And so it goes until we finish the 26 miles at around 2:30 in the afternoon. This has been our routine for more than 100 days. Tomorrow will be the last "normal" day.

**DAY 122.** As I left the motor home to start running in morning darkness, my first thought was, "This is it, my last 26-mile day." Tomorrow will be 18 or 19, and we'll finish with five or so.

Actually, we could finish tomorrow instead of Wednesday without exceeding 26 miles on any day. But we've set 10:00 Wednesday morning as our rendezvous time with friends at the beach.

That means we'll be able to go into the finish relatively fresh and be able to savor every moment of it. A long way we will have come to enjoy those moments.

Second thought early this morning: "Today will put us on our last highway." South Carolina Route 278 will carry us all the way to the beach.

Once on this highway, we no longer needed maps or navigational aids. This is the only road leading onto the island.

We already were within the gravitational pull of Hilton Head Island. Every so often, I saw a sign advertising something in Hilton Head and that pumped a bit of adrenaline. Getting close.

Unfortunately, because Highway 278 leads to a popular vacation area, we ran into a mess of traffic. It set me to worrying, "My God, what a time to get hit with so few miles left!"

I recalled the stories of two marathoners, Dorando Pietri and Jim Peters. Both of them collapsed on the track, only a few yards short of winning major marathons. Caution was my byword for the day.

I had reason to worry. Some sorry driver in a red sports car, passing me from behind, went over the white fog line and missed me by a scant nine inches, even though I'd fled into the weeds. Remembering the earlier incident with the drunk, I exercised remarkable restraint and flashed no gestures.

The day's run complete, Elaine and I drove into Hilton Head to preview our finish and to set up housekeeping on the island. On the way in, we crossed the bridge over the Intercoastal Waterway.

I was relieved to see that the bridge had a breakdown lane. Piece of cake to run this tomorrow. In fact, pleasant miles lay ahead all the way to the Atlantic.

We chose the Motorcoach Resort as our final camping spot. It turned out to be a luxury RV resort with sites privately owned but with some owners renting them.

The setting under an umbrella of pine trees is beautiful and the amenities are many—an Olympic-sized pool, exercise room, sauna, whirlpool, six tennis courts, basketball court, laundromat, and each RV space has its own deck. A fitting spot to celebrate our success, and for only $24 a night.

We quickly solved a logistical problem. We made arrangements with Island Postal Services for my daughter Susan to send our cruise tickets here by Federal Express.

This leaves only the matter of clothes to attend to. We hadn't planned on a cruise when this run began.

Now Elaine and I have to get together a suitable wardrobe for the ship. T-shirts, shorts and jock straps are not going to make it for me, and shoes with toeboxes cut out are hardly fashionable shipboard wear.

This evening, we talk about the two main thoughts on our minds: Only one more morning of getting up early and only two days to go before we could stand in the Atlantic and shout, "My God, we did it!"

**DAY 123.** Elaine has been telling me lately, "I think you're doing too much reminiscing and reflecting in these logs." I reply, "Guilty as charged."

But I remind her that these mental meanderings are a fallout of my disassociating—of purposefully trying to get my mind off running and absorbed in thought. The miles go faster and easier when I can forget how tired or gimpy I am.

To move easier today along the grassy, bumpy, sloped median of the divided road, I said to myself, "We're getting very close to finishing our 3192 miles. The question is, What have we accomplished?"

I came up with these answers:

1. A hidden reward of our run, one we had not anticipated, is that it has brought Elaine and me closer together. We've always had a close relationship. But this RUNXUSA experience has added to this closeness because we worked so harmoniously together, often under adverse circumstances, to reach our goals. We both realize this is something we did together. Along the

way, we shared laughs and disappointments, ups and downs. And when it's over, we will share, as equal partners, the satisfaction of accomplishing what we set out to do.

2. For 20 years, ever since reading *My Run Across the USA* by Don Shepherd, the challenge of a transcon run was on my mind. Could I do it? With Elaine's help, I've met that challenge.

3. Elaine and I were able to meet our goals. We met our goal of averaging 26 miles a day (the final figure will be 26.08). On back roads, we met people and saw places that increased our knowledge of our country and reawakened us to its diversity, its size, its strength. On a vacation of sorts, extending over four months, we injected some excitement and variety into our lives.

4. From the time we started, Elaine was firmly resolved that I would not lose weight. Her nourishment crusade has been successful because I have lost only five pounds to date—less than any other transcon runner has reported.

5. By the grace of God, we were lucky in that: (a) neither of us had any serious illness during the 124 days, though Elaine picked up a toothache that lasted the entire last month; (b) while I had flickers and signals from latent and potential injuries, I incurred no injury that kept me from running; (c) while running, neither of us was attacked by man, beast or car, and (d) our motor home performed well, was comfortable (except when parked roadside during hot days) and wasn't burglarized.

6. Our run is a statement about aging. The very act of running 3192 miles across the country at age 73 will cause some people—old and young—to refocus on aging and physical exercise. Hopefully, some of them will improve their lifestyles, and those already exercise-minded will be reinforced to continue what they are doing. The very fact that a 73-year-old man has run across the USA should be evidence that senior citizens have a greater physical capacity or potential than people generally realize.

7. We remained in action for 124 days, never taking a day off—which, again, is another manifestation that senior citizens have more physical stamina than they are credited with.

When I called my daughter Susan today to tell her where to send our cruise tickets, she excitedly reported, "Herb Caen had an item about your run in his *San Francisco Chronicle* column this morning."

I'm thrilled that a columnist of Caen's stature would

recognize our run. Come to think of it, he is two or three years older than I am and deserves credit for his endurance as a newspaperman.

Tomorrow we get to sleep in! Only tomorrow and our odyssey is over!

**DAY 124.** After all these months of struggling out of bed at 4:30 a.m., lounging there until seven seems almost sinful. At breakfast and driving to the start, Elaine and I are both keyed up, adrenaline pumping over the excitement of this being our last day. But we joke, "It's not over until the fat lady sings!"

This day is purely ceremonial. Media people, contacted by our friends in Savannah, want to meet us at the finish at the appointed time. The only way we could accommodate them for certain was to plan a short day.

From yesterday's reconnaissance, Elaine and I know that the distance to the finish is only 5.2 miles, so this will be a leisurely jaunt with just two concerns along the way: get to the finish safely and at 10 a.m.

Shortly before 8:30, we're in a festive mood as Elaine camcords my final departure. We agree that I'll run three miles to our last pit stop.

The thought that keeps running through my head—as it often has the past few days—is, "I can't believe that we really did it." That thought and the feeling of overwhelming gratitude for being able to do it.

I mutter another prayer of thanks. How many hundred does that make?

It's coming to an end and we're glad it's over. Yet deep inside me is some regret at seeing the curtain come down on this drama I've been enjoying.

Our pit stop is a short one because Elaine will need time to find a parking space near the beach where we finish. Folly Field Beach is now little more than two miles away.

My problems are reduced to these two: turn left at Folly Field Road and don't get hit by a car on the way to the finish.

Running now on the highway median strip, I'm staying as far away from cars as possible, taking no chances of getting hit now. I want to hear the fat lady sing!

My spirits are buoyant—it's a beautiful, beautiful world! Especially if I don't miss Folly Field Road and mess things up.

That concern has me reading every street sign intently even though, from our recon of yesterday, I have a good idea of where this road is located. I come to it a little sooner than expected and, with the utmost of caution, cross the highway and head toward the beach.

I look at my watch and see I'm a bit early. So I throttle down with only three-fourths of a mile to go.

Nearing the beach, I spot Elaine standing by a walkway. Two men are beside her, and she introduces them as newspaper reporters Mike Miller of the (Hilton Head) *Island Packet* and Bill Caton of the *Savannah Morning News*.

They suggest that I run across the beach and into the Atlantic to finish before they conduct their interviews. I try to get Elaine to run with me, but she balks, saying, "It's your moment."

I don't feel that way. It's OUR moment. But she is adamant, saying, "I want to camcord the finish."

I struggle across the sand, damn glad that I don't have to run far in it, and into the Atlantic.

Splash! Water never felt so good!

Elaine follows and dips her hands in the Atlantic. "Just wanted to feel it!" she says.

Now, Elaine and I are standing on the beach, answering the many questions of Miller and Caton when a TV reporter from Channel 11, a CBS affiliate, shows up. He asks if I'll run into the ocean again so that he can photograph my "finish."

Actually, I do this a couple of times to get the shot he wants. But Elaine and I know that only her camcorder has my actual finish.

We chat with all three reporters for almost an hour before they depart for other assignments. We're impressed with the interest all three showed in our run and the intelligence of their questions.

Then we drive back to the RV park, thinking we will relax, but are greeted there with an avalanche of messages. Call KAHI radio in our hometown of Auburn, California. Call Associated Press in Charleston, South Carolina. Call the *Sacramento Bee*.

All want interviews, and we finish each of them with a sense of inadequacy. It's so hard to convey our experiences and feelings during the 124 days of the run. The enormity of it overwhelms us.

We're still having trouble comprehending how we did it. How can we describe it to reporters?

In my life, I've found that many difficult things—many trying times—become easier in retrospect than when actually happening. I hope that we didn't succumb to that thinking in the interviews.

We were never sure that injury, illness or accident wouldn't keep us from finishing until we actually ran into the Atlantic. Never was any day, except the two ceremonial days, a piece of cake. Every mile was work, but work enjoyed.

After the reporters left the beach, Elaine and I stood at the ocean's edge with arms around each other, enjoying the water splashing over our feet. We were silent awhile, then I asked, "What are you thinking?"

Without any hesitation, she said, "That it's over,—and yet that it will never really be over. It's something that will always be with us, as part of us—just yours and mine."

I nodded an affirmative, then Elaine said, "Now tell me what you're thinking."

"Well, I don't know if I can express it. But I've been asking myself how we were able to do it. And I've sort of decided we did it because we controlled our own destiny. "We lived by what we did—or what we failed to do. We were accountable only to ourselves. No board, no CEO, no president, no general, no boss told us what to do and what not to do. We marched to the beat of our own drummer. And also we were able to do it because we were lucky."

Hugging me, Elaine said, "And don't forget God. We both prayed a lot."

"We sure did," I replied, "and God smiled on us."

As we walked off the beach, both of us could hear the fat lady singing.

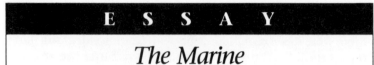

# The Marine
by Frank Bacon

(I introduced Frank, my Marine Corps buddy, when he met us on the road in Georgia. See Days 115 to 117.)

When I went looking for our geriatric gadabout, Paul Reese, that morning in early August 1990 in middle Georgia, I reflected on my comfort in the air-conditioned car as I rode along for our rendezvous in the countryside. Then I empathized with Paul, who must be perspiring freely in the sultry morning air as he trudged on road-weary feet to meet his daily quota of miles.

To my companion in the car, my younger brother Paul, I confided my concerns about how well Paul's reasoning faculties might have survived the passage of 73 years and the many grueling miles—in grinding increments of 26, 50 and even 100 miles—that he had covered in so many parts of the world. I had run cross-country in college, but that was only a small fraction of the distances he ran and, more significantly, 50 years ago.

I recounted to my brother the beginning of my shared Marine Corps experience with Paul Reese. Although he and I were alphabetically segregated into different companies while training for service during World War II, we did share—along with 400 other trainees—the same barracks, the same food, the same early morning runs through the northern Virginia winter in our undershirts, the same boring classroom lectures, the same training hikes and field exercises in the Virginia countryside and the same chilly landing exercises in the Potomac River.

The attack on Pearl Harbor while we were in the midst of this training came as a rude awakening of what lay ahead for us. After the training was over, we second lieutenants went our separate ways.

Years later, in 1978, a couple of us were talking about the "good old days" and decided that it might still be possible to relive some of those days. We located as many of our classmates as possible and scheduled a reunion in New Orleans.

This became an annual event and was moved around the country. Each reunion proved to be better than the previous ones. Our spouses were an integral part of the gatherings, and much planning was done to be sure that they continued to share our enthusiasm.

As I searched for the wayfaring Reeses along the Georgia roads—retracing the route a couple of times—I mused about the strange paths that our lives had taken and how they had converged so satisfyingly in our later years.

Up ahead, about three miles out of Greensboro, Georgia, we saw an RV pulled over to the side of the road. As we slowed, I could read the "RUNXUSA" tag on the front and knew that we had made contact.

Paul was taking one of his breaks, and Elaine had fixed him a high-energy snack to sustain him through the next leg of his daily marathon run. They were both dressed appropriately for the occasion in shorts and T-shirts, and allowed me to take pictures of them for our 7th ROC newsletter.

At dinner the next night, my wife Margie and I told them that some of our classmates in the region wanted to celebrate the conclusion of their remarkable feat with a dinner in Savannah and another luncheon the next day. More importantly, we wanted to assure Paul and Elaine that such a feat would not go unnoted by the general public.

After all, not every 73-year-old is going to be interested in leaving his favorite easy chair to run from the Pacific to the Atlantic. But he would like to read about someone else who was so inclined.

Paul liked the dinner and luncheon ideas. But he was not too keen on the publicity. However, after some encouragement he did agree to it.

When Paul splashed into the Atlantic Ocean at Hilton Head, his classmates were represented by Joe and Judy Hall. Joe had done a splendid job PRing Paul's accomplishment with the local media. He made the evening TV news and rated front-page stories in the Savannah, Hilton Head and Beaufort newspapers.

Two months later, the 7th ROC held its annual reunion in San Francisco. Paul's classmates gave him a standing ovation.

# Epilogue

FALL,1992. As I write this page, two years have passed since RUNXUSA ended. Let me quickly catch you up on what has happened to us in the meantime.

The Savannah festivities concluded, our next move was to fly to Miami and board the Nordic Empress for a five-day Caribbean cruise—the big payday (as if I really could repay her) for Elaine's pit-crewing. Because my daughter Susan and her husband, Ed Granlund, had made several journeys from the Bay Area to Auburn (about 250 miles round-trip) to look after our home and pay our bills, we invited them to accompany us.

Following the cruise, Elaine and I returned to Savannah and the motor home—only to find it had been invaded by a colony of ants. After exterminating them, we left on a leisurely drive home, plotting a route that would not retrace any of our eastward journey. Compared to what we had been through coming east at 26 miles a day, covering close to 300 miles daily while returning seemed overwhelmingly fast.

On September 14, 1990, we arrived back home in Auburn, California, after having been away 148 days. Elaine, never one to waste time, collected four days later on her promise from me. I handed a kennel owner a check, and he handed Elaine a five-week-old black Labrador whom we promptly named Rebel.

About five months later, Elaine suddenly decided, by what stretch of logic I know not, that Rebel was lonesome and needed a companion. Brudder, a two-month-old brown Lab, entered our family.

Both mutts have contributed much happiness and health to Elaine, since she walks them three miles almost every day. I admit to enjoying both critters, too, even though parenting these youngsters is not easy for a guy in his mid-70s.

I'm not racing as frequently or as fast as I did before going across the country, and neither is George Billingsley. George and I still run together a couple of times a week, and we're both trying to figure out why we're dragging in speed and endurance.

Did RUNXUSA drain us? Certainly our losses can't be attributable to age. Gosh, I'm only 75, and George is a 70-year-old kid.

I've reached my 75th birthday in good health. Regular tests have shown no sign of the prostate cancer for which I was treated five years ago.

I took this old body into the shop right after the transcon run, and two different doctors pronounced me none the worse for wear orthopedically. The first was Loren Blickenstaff, M.D. My daughter-in-law, Kathy Blume, a surgical nurse, had arranged for me to see him in Boise on our trip home.

Orthopedist Blickenstaff commented, "I examined the hips and knees of Mr. Reese after his run across the United States and found them to be surprisingly normal. The surrounding bone was of excellent quality. One would be unable to differentiate between his X-rays and those of a normal 30-year-old male."

On returning home, I visited orthopedist Gilbert Lang, M.D., in Roseville, California. He performed a magnetic resonance imaging exam, compared it with a previous MRI and concluded, "There was no appreciable change noted between the two studies."

Dr. Lang added, "I felt prior to the run that the chances of the [left, recently injured] knee holding up for that prolonged time period without any rest periods would be small. Fortunately, I was proven wrong.

"From an orthopedic standpoint, this would have been a very significant accomplishment in a young person. For somebody with this many years and miles on his equipment, it was a spectacular accomplishment."

This fall, Elaine and I returned to Hilton Head Island—by plane this time for the annual reunion with my Marine Corps classmates. We crossed the sandy beach, splashed into the Atlantic and relived the jubilant moment of two years ago.

I'd said then that it was an experience I wouldn't trade for a fortune or repeat for a fortune. Elaine had agreed at the time.

Then she took me completely by surprise me one day in mid-1992 when she said, "I'd like to try another adventure run. But I've got a couple of conditions. First, we take the dogs. Second, you limit the scope of the run to two or three weeks."

I liked the idea and added a condition of my own. To spare my weary body parts and allow for more recreational time, I'd limit my daily distance to 20 miles.

I hit upon the goal of running across all the western states. On short notice, I squeezed in Oregon this September.

I'd already done California, Nevada, Utah and Colorado. Now my battle plan is to work in the other six—Arizona, New Mexico, Washington, Idaho, Montana and Wyoming—within the next three years.

One of the secrets of aging gracefully is always to have something to look forward to. Onward to those other western states!

# *Appendix 1*

## BESTS AND WORSTS

Here's my list of superlatives from 124 days on America's roads:

## BESTS

| | |
|---|---|
| Most colorful town | Austin, Nevada |
| Best state for scenery | Colorado |
| Thickest forestation | Georgia |
| Most pleasant small towns | Delta, Co., and Tribune, Ks. |
| Friendliest people | Utah and Kansas |
| Most efficient Highway Patrol | Utah |
| Best restaurant | Jailhouse in Ely, Nevada |
| Most considerate drivers | Utah |
| Biggest surprise | so many mountains (eight) over 6000 feet in Nevada |
| Best sunrises and sunsets | Nevada and Utah deserts |
| Best state parks | Georgia |
| Best backroad | abandoned Highway 50 in Utah and Colorado |
| Best RV park | Motorcoach Resort, Hilton Head Island |
| Best small-town park | Coffeyville, Kansas |
| Most considerate farmer | Irish Anderson of Delta, Ut. |
| Best of hundreds of dogs | Mr. McGillicuddy |
| Most humorous incident | (1) George leaving motor home and heading west instead of east |

## WORSTS

| | |
|---|---|
| Most depressing city | Pueblo, Colorado |
| Most depressing small town | Cotton Plant, Arkansas |
| Most discourteous drivers | Colorado |
| Most litter | Mississippi |
| Most unfriendly people | Oklahoma |
| Most annoying experience | being bitten by hordes of flies in Kansas |
| Foulest odor | rendering plant in Kansas |
| Most pathetic sight | cottontail in Leoti, Kansas, gasping for each breath in 108-degree heat |

# *Appendix 2*

## RECORD CROSSINGS

In his book *Ultramarathon,* James E. Shapiro lists the progressive records for runs across the USA. He points out that the length of routes differs and that proof of the runner actually covering the entire distance on foot wasn't required. Here is Shapiro's listing:

| Name | Year | Time | Distance | Route |
|---|---|---|---|---|
| John Ennis | 1890 | 80.2 days | unknown | NYC-SF |
| Edward Weston | 1910 | 77 days | 3483m | NYC-LA |
| James Hocking | 1924 | 75 days | 3754m | SF-NYC |
| Don Shepherd | 1964 | 73.3 days | 3200m | LA-NYC |
| Bruce Tulloh | 1969 | 64.9 days | 2876m | LA-NYC |
| Marvin Swigart | 1971 | 62.7 days | 3266m | SF-NYC |
| John Bull | 1972 | 53.9 days | 2876m | LA-NYC |
| E. Gordon Brooks | 1974 | 53.3 days | 2876m | NYC-LA |
| Tom McGrath | 1977 | 53.0 days | 3046m | NYC-SF |

Omitted is Abraham Lincoln Monteverde, who at age 61 in 1920 ran across the USA (New York City to San Francisco) in 79 days. Since publication of Shapiro's book, Frank Giannino Jr. has claimed the record by running 3100 miles from San Francisco to New York City in 46 days, eight hours.

**WOMEN'S RECORD**

| | | | | |
|---|---|---|---|---|
| Mavis Hutchinson | 1978 | 69.9 days | 2871m | LA-NYC |

**WALKING RECORD**

| | | | | |
|---|---|---|---|---|
| John Lees | 1972 | 53.5 days | 2876m | LA-NYC |

**OLDEST WOMAN**

| | | | | |
|---|---|---|---|---|
| Annabel Marsh | 1984 | 126 days | 3200m | SF-DC |

**OLDEST MAN**

| | | | | |
|---|---|---|---|---|
| Paul Reese | 1990 | 124 days | 3192m | Jenner-HHI |

# *Appendix 3*

## ADVICE ON RUNNING TOURING

One surprising aftermath of my run has been the number of runners writing to ask for advice on undertaking such adventures. I soon realized that many more people would be running across the country if they were not shackled with the necessity of earning a living. Most of those inquiring said they had the project on hold until they could afford the time and money to do it.

But wait a minute, I found myself thinking. In the meantime, there is a way out for these runners. What they can do NOW is some type of multiday run—say from one town to another, one national park to another, one landmark to another, one state border to another. These can be runs of any duration, a few days to a couple of weeks, depending on the vacation time available.

Thinking of this, I decided to package the advice so that it will have twofold application: First, it will guide anyone planning a transcon run. Second, it will be helpful to anyone planning a multiday run. That said, here are 25 suggestions.

1. The basic consideration when setting out on a run of this type is that you take the time and effort to enjoy it. If your only desire is to complete the run as fast as possible, see nothing along the way, take the shortest route, ignore people, you might as well stick with road races.

2. Set a realistic daily goal in miles, and try to tie this in with some recreational time. My goal was not less than 25 nor more than 27 miles a day. My average turned out to be 26.08.

3. Plan your attack before starting. How are you going to get your mileage for each day? Three possible systems are: Run continuously, split mileage into two legs, or use three legs. To illustrate, say your goal is 30 miles a day. Continuously, you would start, make your planned pit stops and keep going until you reach 30. With two splits, you would run 15 in the morning, rest, then do 15 in the afternoon. With three splits, the day would break into three 10-mile legs.

4. From the beginning, realize there will be no easy days. You will have road problems, traffic problems, weather problems, logistical problems and more.

5. Nothing is more critical to the runner's enjoyment and success

than his or her pit-crew, whether that be one person or several people. It is imperative that the runner and pit-crew are 100-percent compatible. You are a team. Work out a standard operating procedure so that each will know where they stand at all times.

6. A word about support vehicles: A motor home is ideal, but it should not be more than 20 to 22 feet because a bigger one is too difficult to park for the many required pit stops. A van would be second-best, followed by a station wagon.

7. A pit-crew is imperative for a transcon run. While it's also preferable for a multiday run, it isn't a requirement if there is more than one runner. Two or more runners can leapfrog their cars over the course each day. By that, I mean they could leave one car at the finish, drive back to the start in another car while leaving supplies along the route, then return for the starting-line car later.

8. Don't underestimate or underplan logistical considerations. As an example, I ran 3192 miles across the country. At the same time, Elaine drove 7000 miles pit-crewing for me and attending to our logistical needs.

9. No matter how precise your planning, there will be unexpected happenings—such as a road detour. Be prepared to to handle the unexpected.

10. Carry at least two, preferably three, types of maps for each state—such as AAA, Rand McNally and an official state highway map—because no single map is complete or adequate.

11. In your planning, try to think of any gear or equipment you may need and bring it. For example, on the desert and despite my use of Blistex, my lips chapped and bled. I bought a bandanna, wore it a few days, and my lips healed. Carry a well-stocked medical kit.

12. While on the road, it's unlikely that you will have the chance to buy shoes. So pamper yourself with an adequate supply. On a transcon run, your shoe size will increase. Mine did by one-half size for each 1000 miles. Even on a multiday run, it would be smart to carry one pair of shoes a half-size larger than you normally wear.

13. Keep yourself well stoked with food and drink at each pit stop. This nourishment is vital for keeping up your strength and maintaining your weight.

14. Maintain a regular schedule to make body adaptation easier. And get sufficient sleep, a must for recuperation.

15. Your biggest problem most likely will be finding running space on the road. Roads are made for cars, not runners. Roads

with bike lanes are your best bet.

16. Plan your routing to avoid metropolitan complexes and their environs. My three most miserable days on the road were when I was within 40 miles of Atlanta, Georgia.

17. Before starting, have a clear understanding that there is much inherent danger in the run—danger of your being hit by a car or your support vehicle being in an accident. Be ever alert and cautious. This may sound facetious, but have a good life-insurance policy and make sure your will is in order.

18. Before you leave on a transcon run, have a general delivery post office address for one city in each state, along with the zip code of that address, and give these addresses to those who want to communicate with you. On a multiday run, where mail might not catch up with you, establish phone numbers where messages can be left for you.

19. Take one day at a time. Enjoy it, survive it. If your experience is like mine, in time you will think of just going from one pit stop to the next instead of one day to the next.

20. Associate. Constantly monitor your body. Assess for potential injuries. Take all preventive measures.

21. Disassociate. Get your mind off running and onto other things. If you can "space out" this way, time and miles will pass easier.

22. Maintain and exercise your sense of humor. You will have your ups and downs, but your psyche should remain constant. By that, I mean upbeat.

23. Believe you can do it. Think no other way but "Yes, I can." The human body is capable of considerably more physical endurance than most of us realize.

24. Regardless of whether your run is transcon or multiday, keep a diary with each day's observations. This helps you to put the experience into perspective, to absorb it and to rekindle it later.

25. Observe and appreciate. Drink in the sunrise and sunset, watch a horse cavort, study a beautiful tree, enjoy majestic colors, communicate with people, and thank God daily for the body to do this run. And pray, too, that God will smile on you. You will need that and a lot of luck.

# A MESSAGE FROM THE PUBLISHER

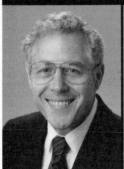

*After I read Paul Reese's manuscript, I made arrangements to meet him in our San Francisco office, as I not only wanted to see a 73-year-old guy capable of running a marathon a day for 124 days, but wanted to actually take a jog with him. I told Paul that my main impression from reading his story was that he made it sound so easy I thought I could do it. Paul said, "That's exactly what I wanted to do. The secret is just in doing it."*

**W. R. Spence, M.D.**
**Publisher**

*T*he book division of WRS Publishing focuses on true stories about everyday heroes, like Paul Reese, who have accomplished their own impossible dreams. While it is sometimes easy to turn a profit with stories of greed, sex, and violence, we are not interested in such books. We only produce books we can be proud of and that can change lives for the better. **Call us at 1-800-299-3366 for suggestions or for a free book catalog.**

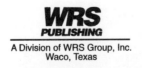

**WRS**
**PUBLISHING**

A Division of WRS Group, Inc.
Waco, Texas

# THE

# RED BADGE OF COURAGE

## And Other Writings

▣▣▣

RIVERSIDE EDITIONS

RIVERSIDE EDITIONS

UNDER THE GENERAL EDITORSHIP OF

*Gordon N. Ray*